Snippets of a Vet's Life

The Early Years

By Rod Graham

With Andrew Jefferis

Illustrations by Veronica Oborn Jefferis

Dedication

To Max and Anne

"Wager"

Dr Hugh Forbes

and

my Children/Grandchildren

for whom Snippets were written

Published by Snippets Press

2025

Snippets of a Vet's Life: The Early Years © 2025
Rod Graham

All rights reserved.

No part of this publication may be reproduced, stored in a retrieval system, or transmitted in any form or by any means, electronic, mechanical, photocopying, recording, or otherwise, without prior written permission from the author, except for brief quotations used in reviews or critical articles.

This is a work of fiction. While inspired by real events, names, characters, and incidents are products of the author's imagination or are used fictitiously. Any resemblance to actual persons, living or dead, is entirely coincidental.

First published in Australia by **Snippets Press**
www.vetsnippets.com.au

Cover design © Snippets Press

Edited by Andrew Jefferis

Made in Australia

V: 18/12/2025-M#1

PREFACE

The Author's Dilemma

Being a veterinarian involves seeing people in times that they rarely share with others. Over the years, when I've had their animals in my care, I have also experienced the owners' hopes, worries, fear, and secrets. And unconsciously, their stories have been archived in my memory.

Add I repeat, *their* stories.

To bring these stories to light, raises an ethical and moral question: how can I reveal their stories while remembering they are not truly mine to tell?

For me, the answer is to reveal the essence rather than the exact events, the feelings, the lessons, the humour, and all the things that make a vet's life what it is, but without revealing the real lives, and the real facts behind the stories.

Snippets of a Vet's Life is a collection of vignettes inspired by truth, but not bound to it. It's not about concealing the truth. It's about preserving it. The Coldstream Veterinary Clinic, the local Coldstream hospital, and Emmerton House are fictional entities that exist only within the pages of the book. Names have been changed, and even in those stories closely related to my own adventures, the details have been altered.

Dr Rob McBride, does not exist, and he is not me, but his experiences and reactions are the experiences and reactions of many young vets.

As Marcel Proust wrote, "Remembrance of things past is not necessarily the remembrance of things as they were."

What you'll read here is memory at work: part fact, part feeling, all shaped by time and experience.

They are my memories, and mine alone.

njoy.

Rod Graham
At my desk.
In my clinic
Melbourne 2025

INTRODUCTION

THE TOUR GUIDE

I was in Bali for a veterinary conference, but in reality, it was a glorified junket.

Each day, after morning lectures, three buses arrived at our hotel to take us on another tour. On the last day, and after a boozy lunch, we were sitting in the bus, while waiting to start the trip back to the hotel. Many of us were rowdy and a few, loquacious.

One vet, in particular, was very drunk. He was loud and sitting next to me. I had got to know him over the last few days, and he was a good guy. But drunk, he became a different person. He could be very rude to people, especially if they were in a *lesser* role.

It was he who asked the question.

Each day, an older Balinese man stood at the front of the bus. He was there to help us at our various destinations, and to be honest, at times, one or two of us had been a bit dismissive of him. For much of our daily journeys, he stood quietly at the front, serenely gazing over this rowdy group of Australian veterinarians.

He always had a gentle smile, no matter what we did or said. And on the last day, my drunk friend, for no apparent reason, suddenly stood up, lurched and addressed, in a somewhat rude manner, our Balinese guide:

'Hey, mate! Why are you always SO BLOODY HAPPY?'

The guide maintained his benign smile and answered him quietly. What he said quickly brought silence to the bus and even to my drunk friend, and we all knew that we had just heard something... profound.

'I am Balinese, and we believe that you are what I am. If I am angry, you are angry. If I am happy, you are happy. If I am sad, you are sad. I choose to be happy so that you, too, can be happy.'

Silence.

He stood, still smiling, but now we could all see that there was also a quiet dignity about his presence. The bus started, and the short trip back to the hotel continued in muted conversation, and my drunken friend slept.

I could not get the tour guide's wisdom out of my head, and in fact, years later, I still use it as an overriding paradigm of behaviour in my own veterinary practice, both to my fellow workers and to our clients:

'You Are, What I Am.'

But... I didn't always have this wisdom....

Table of Contents

1 – AN OLD LADY IN NEED..1
2 – THE COLD CALL TO COLDSTREAM......................................10
3 – SLEEPING IN THE DOG HOUSE..20
4 – THE MATRON AND MR BROWN..27
5 – UP CLOSE AND PERSONAL WITH A MARE.........................35
6 – THE GOAT...42
7 – THE GREEN COTTAGE..53
8 – THE MATRON'S GIFT..62
9 – IN THE DEEP END...73
10 – A NIGHT AT THE OPERA...81
11 – ONE PLUS TWO DEATHS..89
12 – HILLARY AND HANNAH THE HEN......................................98
13 – MRS PRIDHAM'S CLOCK...107
14 – A CLIENT COMPLAINS...113
15 – WE ARE HERE TO HELP YOU, MADAM.............................126
16 – AN EVENING NEVER TO BE FORGOTTEN.........................135
17 – TEDDY AND TETANUS..141
18 – GETTING DOWN TO BUSINESS...155
19 – A ROOSTER, A DONKEY, AND A PAIR OF SPEEDOS.......164
20 – THANK YOU FOR YOUR SERVICE, MAX..........................176
21 – MEETING BOS..182
22 – LIFE'S A LOTTERY...191
23 – A COW SUDDENLY DIES...198
24 – ORAL EXAMS, IN PARTICULAR: COWS............................207
25 – THE FAVOURITE..212
26 – ENTER COLUMBINA, STAGE LEFT.....................................219

27 – THE MOTHER OF ALL HOLIDAYS..228
28 – WAGER: WHO LET THE HOUND IN?..................................234
29 – A DESPERATE NIGHT CALL..242
30 – WHEN A MAN LOSES HIS MATE.......................................248
31 – WHEN A BOY LOSES HIS MATE..257
32 – AN UNEXPECTED VISITOR...264
33 – ACTING THE GOAT WITH A ROOSTER............................268
34 – LUCY'S LAST LIGHT..276
35 – THE STITCH UP AND THE SECRET..................................287
36 – THE DRUNK NEIGHBOUR..292
37 – THE PURVEYOR OF DREAMS..297
38 – A COLLEAGUE AND A COW IN NEED...............................304
39 – CHADWICK AND CO..310
40 – THREE LEGS, TWO FRIENDS AND ONE GOAT..................317
41 – DINNER AT THE GREEN COTTAGE..................................323
42 – THE CUT THAT DIDN'T GO TO PLAN...............................332
43 – ONE CHRISTMAS EVE..340
44 – A SNAKE IN THE GRASS..351
45 – THE PURSUIT OF HAPPINESS...359
46 – THE LAST CALL...371
Epilogue..381

Snippets of a Vet's Life

1 – AN OLD LADY IN NEED

'I don't want to alarm you, but it just may be rabies.'

And I could see in the light of the battery lamp that her face went white.

Rabies is a deadly viral disease that humans can catch and die from, if bitten by an infected dog or other infected species. For good reason, the old name for Rabies was *hydrophobia*, reflecting the excessive salivation of infected dogs, which resulted from their inability to drink.

There is no cure.

I was on weekend duty not long after I had started work as a newly minted veterinarian. I was relieved that I now had a base, a cottage to call home, and no longer needed to sleep on a camp stretcher in the kennel room at the Coldstream Vet Clinic, and in the same room as the occasional complaining dog. I now had my own bed, of sorts: a mattress on the kitchen floor of a rundown weatherboard abode quaintly called The Green Cottage.

Rod Graham

Before leaving the clinic that Saturday afternoon, I had left a now familiar message on the answering machine.

'The Coldstream Veterinary Clinic is now closed. For urgent after-hours assistance, please call... ' and I gave my home phone number.

As the weeks progressed, I noticed that, at times, I began to accentuate the word 'urgent'.

My employer was fair, and we shared the after-hours duty. One night ON, one night OFF, one weekend ON, next weekend OFF. Somebody was always available to help. Being 'on Call' to 'help' meant that whoever was on duty that night or the weekend was tied to their home phone and had to stay at home or, in some way, be contactable. It was a time before mobile phones and just before personal pagers became economically available to vets.

Because I lived alone, in the Green Cottage, whenever I was out on a call, I would switch on my home 'answer phone', encouraging whoever had rung to leave a message so that I could call them back when I returned. Answer machines were a precursor to the ubiquitous voicemail on our smartphones, and on this night, after I had returned from stitching a horse's leg cut in a barbed wire fence, I noticed the machine's red light blinked as I entered the kitchen. Somebody had left a message.

It was 10:30 pm, and I needed sleep.

Snippets of a Vet's Life

I pressed the green replay button. Her voice was frail, and she sounded very distressed.

'Hello. Hello. Are you there? Could you help me? My dog has gone mad, and I have locked him in our garden room. Can you call me?'

And I did.

She lived in Yarra Glen, about 5 km from my home. I drove quickly and, using a map, found Valley View Rd. Her directions were good, and I promptly located her house and knocked on the front door. The hall light went on, and a short, older lady cautiously opened the door.

She was slightly bent, which made her appear much smaller than I was. With a slight upward tilt of her head, her grey hair covered in part by a scarf, she addressed me with an urgent, wispy voice, 'Yes?'

'Hi, Mrs Denham,' I said quietly as I looked down at her upturned face, adding, ' I'm... Dr Rob, the vet. You called...?

I turned slightly to one side as if to leave in case I had misunderstood the directions and was at the wrong house. I was still getting used to using and saying the word 'Dr.' before my name.

Then, with a stronger voice, I continued, 'I'm the vet you called...,' but I still wondered if it was the wrong house.

'Oh, I'm sorry. It's just that you look so young, dear,' she said and then continued, 'Come in and thank you for coming.' She abruptly turned, walking away from me along the inside passage. I hesitated. Should I follow? I was uncertain.

She looked back towards me and said, 'This way, dear. Outside in the back garden shed.'

She led the way through her home, out the back door, and along a path to a small wooden outbuilding. From inside, I could hear the sound of a dog, sounding angrier as we approached.

'There are no lights out here, but I have a lamp. Will that do?'

'Yes. Now tell me again what happened?'

'Well, dear, Benjamin is my late husband's dog. And since he passed away, Benji and I have grown closer. But this week, for the first time, Benji growled at me when I went to get him off the couch.'

'I see. What type of dog is Benjamin?'

'He's a Border Collie. He's always been a nice dog and has never growled at anybody. But this week... he's been different. And tonight, he did something unusual. He put himself in the garden shed, and has been barking, as if he's gone ... mad?'

'What then happened?'

'Well, dear, I called him for his dinner. He loves dinner. But he didn't come. I found him curled up on a mat in the shed. I bent down to take his collar. He pulled back and snarled at me. He looked different. It was as though he didn't recognise me.'

'I see. Yes, very strange,' I agreed while wondering what was happening with the much loved Benjamin.

He sounded like he had, for some reason, an irritated central nervous system and had lost some of his inherent behavioural controls, which are centred in the frontal lobes of his brain. It is very similar to a person with a head injury. They can become aggressive, irrational, and irritable. I raked my university educated but inexperienced brain for possible causes of a dog's relatively sudden onset of aggression or mania. Poisoning, drugs, encephalitis, head injury? I was perplexed, and then I remembered a lecture about a cow in Thailand that had suddenly become aggressive to the local villagers, and a postmortem examination revealed the cause of its behaviour change was rabies.

Was this rabies?

I knew that Australia was free of this ancient malady and that our livestock industry relied on its absence for the continued prosperity of our Live Animal Export trade. But what if the virus had somehow breached our bio-security and made its way to Yarra Glen?

What if Benjamin had contracted the virus? And worse, what if I *missed* it? That was my biggest fear. My *mistake* could wreck the Australian agricultural economy. This may sound far-fetched, but this is ALL young vets fear: that they will miss *something really important*!

So that is why I said, 'I don't wish to alarm you, Mrs Denham, but Benjamin may have rabies,' which did cause her to be alarmed.

I quickly added, 'But it may not be... I'm unsure. Maybe... I could... make a phone call?'

'Yes, dear. This way.'

I wasn't entirely comfortable with being called 'dear'; it seemed to detract from my new elevated status of veterinarian. In reality, I wasn't comfortable either with the honorary title Doctor that the professional body, the Australian Veterinary Association had, a few years earlier, bestowed upon veterinarians in Victoria.

'There's the phone, dear...Benji is going to be alright, isn't he?'

I smiled weakly to acknowledge her concern as I dialled my boss's home number. 'Hello,' he answered with a drowsy voice.

'Doug. Sorry to disturb your sleep. Got this dog in Yarra Glen. She's a new client, so I don't know much about her. I don't think the dog has been to a vet for a while, if ever.'

I had not yet examined Benjamin or, for that matter, even seen him. Doug listened as I described the symptoms, and I did say that I was a bit worried.

'OK. Robbie. Were you wondering if it had rabies?'

Snippets of a Vet's Life

'Yes. I was Doug. How did you know?'

'Been there myself when I had just graduated,' he said, adding, 'It sounds like the neurological complication of untreated distemper. We don't often see it now, but I bet that is what it is. All you can do is put the dog down. Nothing else you can do.'

'Thanks,' I said, putting the phone down. I passed on the revised diagnosis to relieve Mrs Denham, whose face lit up joyfully.

But it was to be short-lived. I was young and not well-versed in giving confrontational messages. And so, on seeing her smile, I quickly added that I could do nothing to treat Benjamin except put him 'out of his misery.'

'But he's my husband's dog! I promised him I would take care of Benjamin.'

'It's the only thing I'm afraid...'

'I can't....' She looked at me, and I remained silent, just looking back at her, giving her time to process what I had said and what I had told her we needed to do.

'And there is nothing you can do,' she pleaded.

'Nothing.'

Her lower lip quivered as she quietly said, 'OK, do it,' and left the room.

I stood outside the garden shed door. Benjamin was still growling inside. I gently eased the door slightly open, just enough to allow me to assess the situation and, if necessary, quickly shut it to prevent his escape or, worse, attack.

But there was no lunging at the open doorway as I had feared. Benjamin did not move but continued to growl. I opened the door further and went in.

He was growling and, at times, biting at things in the air. He took little notice of me. But then he turned his head toward me. The movement caused his neck to twitch, and he fell to the floor. He was clearly in a 'bad' way.

Even though he was on the floor and struggling to get up, he still growled. I looked about the little shed and saw a large canvas garden bag hanging on the wall. I grabbed at it and threw it over Benjamin's head, and, with my left knee, and as gently as I could, I pinned him to the floor and then injected a strong anaesthetic drug into his thigh muscle. I knew it was not the best way of administering the drug to end his life. It would be painful, but it was the only way to use it in a chaotic situation. I continued to hold him down. He struggled for a few minutes but then gradually relaxed as the barbiturate started to have its anaesthetic effect. He lay under my knee. He got deeper and deeper into the anaesthetic from which he would never wake. I could feel his life coming to an end. I touched the cornea of one of his eyes. There was no response. His brain was dead.

Snippets of a Vet's Life

Mrs Denham waited in the kitchen and quietly asked, 'Is it done?'

'Yes,' I replied.

Her hand went to her face, now suffused with grief.

'Where is he?'

'Still in the shed.'

'Oh, Benjamin. Benji... What will I do with him? I don't know...' and her voice trailed off.

I thought for a minute, considering what I knew about this person that I had recently met: her recent loss of a husband and now the sudden loss of a much loved dog. I was tired. It had been a very long day. I could have just left her, but something made me think of my mother and wonder what help she would need in such a situation.

'Have you got a shovel or spade, Mrs. Denham?'

And together we buried Benjamin. As I made my way back to the Green Cottage, I reflected that Doug was a good boss, a good mentor and I was grateful for his steady guidance in this case. I stretched out for a much needed sleep on the kitchen floor.

But sleeping on that floor was never the work of chance or accident. To see how I came to be there, the clock must be turned back a few short weeks, to my final year at university, when the hunt for jobs was on, yet such positions were as rare as hen's teeth, and even harder to find because I wanted to be a horse vet.

2 – THE COLD CALL TO COLDSTREAM

It was the eve of my final year, a season of endings and new beginnings. We were still students, but barely. The edges of our white clinic coats were sometimes soiled, our debts growing, our anxieties increasing, and for many of us, our futures still hazy like morning fog before sunrise.

We were approaching the final examinations and the void that lay beyond.

But, earlier that year, in the student dining hall, a confident young man, a few years older than most of us, stood up and demanded our attention.

Tony was neither a doctor nor a dentist, nor a surgeon nor a scholar. He was an accountant, fresh-faced, bright-eyed, with the energy of someone who had recently discovered his own usefulness. Instead of surgical gowns or a stethoscope, he carried spreadsheets in his mind and business cards in his pocket. A few years earlier, Tony had started an accounting practice with his brother, focusing on the financial needs of doctors, dentists, and veterinarians. To attract clients, he pitched to us, the graduating class, at a dinner shortly after my final year began. He presented on financial management for veterinarians, and during his talk, I learned he was looking for a student to serve as their veterinary student representative.

This got my attention.

After dinner, I made my way toward Tony. I waited while one or two other students asked questions, and then it was my turn. I stepped toward him and extended my hand.

'Hi, Tony. I'm Rob. Great talk. Thanks. Really interesting,' but it was not exactly the truth.

'Rob!' and he vigorously shook my hand. 'Good to meet you.' He looked intently at me with a welcoming smile. He had a vibrancy and enthusiasm about him, and he gave the feeling that he was always in a rush.

'One question. What's involved in being the local student representative?'

'Good, good...good, Rob. Now, the representative position...' He paused, gathering his thoughts. 'All you have to do is keep us informed about what's happening with the student body. There's no pay, but once you graduate, we can help you at the start of your career.'

'What sort of help?'

'Well, for example, if you need a job, we have contacts through our clients and can help you find one.'

Even at this stage of my career, I recognised the value of networking.

'OK. Sounds good. I probably won't need help, as I'll be returning interstate, but I'm happy to give it a try. Let's see what happens.'

'Great, Rob. Here's my card.'

Later that year, once the thrill of graduation had given way to the more sobering question of employment, I realised I was in need of a helping hand. Circumstances, as they so often do, conspired to leave me standing without a clear direction. It was then, with a touch of sheepishness, that I turned to Tony. He had the kind of connections and quiet wisdom that opened doors, and in that moment, I found myself grateful, and just a little amused, at how quickly youthful independence can give way to the need for help.

A sultry female voice answered the phone.

'How can I help you?'

'Can I speak with Tony, please?'

'Is he expecting your call?'

I paused to consider my response.

'Sort of...'

'I'll put you through.'

Snippets of a Vet's Life

'Yes. Hello. Tony here,' he said in a rapid staccato. 'Hello.'

'Hi, Tony. Rob McBride here. I'm your year rep for the vets.'

'Yes! Of course, Rob… Um.' There was a short silence, probably as he recalled who I was. 'Rob! Yes, how can I help you?'

Tony always spoke with great enthusiasm, and as though he had a smile on his face.

'Well, Tony, things are a bit light in the job market for young horse vets, and I need a job. You said to call if I needed help. Hence my phone call.'

'I see. Yes.'

I felt the smile leave his face.

'There aren't many jobs currently available, but let's see what I can do for you. Can you come to my office next Tuesday at about 1:30 pm?'

'Yes.'

He gave me the address, and our telephone call ended.

A few days later, I was nervous as I ascended the stairs to the first floor of Tony's accountancy office, on the outskirts of the city's business district. After hesitantly introducing myself to the receptionist, who, looking nothing like her telephone voice, pushed a button, and a door opened. Tony appeared. He had a big smile as he extended his arm and greeted me with a vigorous handshake.

'Rob. Good to see you. Come in, come in. This way…'

He was welcoming and directed me to a chair on one side of a large desk. On it was a large plastic pyramid with a telephone dialer at its base and a handset on top. I concluded it was a telephone, but nothing like I had ever seen.

It was the first time I had encountered a 'speaker telephone.'

'OK, Rob, let's get down to getting you a job. I know you want to be a horse vet, but as you've probably found out, there aren't any positions available for new grads in that field currently. Let me be frank. Usually, unless you've made connections as a student to a horse practice, it can be difficult to land a job as a newly graduated vet in equine work. So, my first question for you is: do you have any connections?'

'No. I don't.'

I didn't reveal that I had worked for a barrister during the previous two summer breaks, as I hadn't spent my summer vacations with vets, as expected of a veterinary student.

'Seeing' practice with vets, as I was supposed to do as part of completing my undergraduate degree, didn't pay anything. I was constantly in need of funds to cover my accommodation as a veterinary student.

Snippets of a Vet's Life

Hence, I took a job with a well-paying lawyer, who just happened to be called a doctor. Why? As a PhD graduate in Law, he was entitled to the honorific 'Doctor,' and the job, working on his estate at Mt. Macedon, was well paid.

The vet school never uncovered my little ruse: I was 'seeing' practice with a barrister, not a vet. His only link to veterinary medicine? He was writing a book, Horse and the Law while I mucked out stables at his place in Mt. Macedon.

I didn't see the point in correcting their mistake, but the Universe has a way of repaying dishonesty: I had no horse vet contacts who could give me a job.

Tony remained oblivious to this history, directing me to stay seated as he left the room. A few minutes later, he returned with a folder under his right arm.

'OK, Rob. I'm going to call a vet. His name is Douglas. He's a good vet, a good person, and one of our valued clients. He runs a general veterinary practice in Coldstream, and I know he handles a variety of animals, including horses, cows, as well as dogs and cats. However, he doesn't particularly enjoy doing the horse work so it may give you an opportunity. What do you think?'

I thought for a few seconds and then said,

'OK. I'm in.'

Tony punched a number into the dialer, and after the connection was established, he replaced the handset and continued talking from his seat, hands-free..

Amazing! His use of new technology was very impressive.

'Doug. I've been looking at your financials, and I think it's time you put on a young vet.'

'Are you sure?' said an uncertain voice emanating from the white pyramid on Tony's neat desk.

'Yes, Doug. You can't keep working full-time like you have over the last few years. And I know you want to start a family, so it's time. You can afford to put on a new graduate. And I've got him sitting in front of me. Say hello, Rob.'

'Hi Doug, I'm Rob' I said, directing my voice toward the pyramid telephone.

'Rob. Good to meet you. Listening to Tony, I should give you a job. I'm in Coldstream, and we attend to a mixture of small animals, cows, and horses.'

'Sounds great. I especially want to work with horses.'

'That's good because I prefer cows to horses,' he paused and added, '...and horse owners.'

'That sounds good to me. When would you like me to start, if I'm acceptable to you?'

'What about the 20th of December?'

Snippets of a Vet's Life

That was about two weeks away.

'Sure,' I said, 'but there's one thing. I would probably need a few days off during the Royal Melbourne Show next year to ride a friend's horse in some events. Would that be a problem?'

'No problem. By then, you would have accrued some holiday leave. Any other questions?'

I gave it some thought, but I had no questions. I had never been employed before, except for summer jobs.

'No. I think that's all,' I answered.

'OK. You're employed.'

'Great. That was simple. I do have one other question. I'm not trying to be rude, but...how much do I get paid?'

I was slightly uncomfortable asking about money. Many young vets aren't motivated by salaries, and in this regard, I was no exception. I was just glad that I had a job.

'Award salary, plus on duty every second night, plus on duty every second weekend. You'll be sharing the after-hours calls with me. OK with you?'

'Yes. And do you know what the award is?'

'No. Tony? Do you know?'

'Yep. $10,000 a year, plus four weeks' annual leave. Nothing for after hours.' Tony quickly answered, obviously an answer that was at his fingertips.

For a student in my graduating year, and surviving on $2000 a year, that seemed an enormous amount.

I readily replied,

'Seems fair. That's OK with me. I'm in.'

'OK, Rob. I'll see you in two weeks. Give me a call before you arrive," and he dictated his clinic number. 'Nothing else, Tony?'

'Nothing, Doug. Goodbye,' said Tony, pushing a button at the base of the white pyramid.

He stood up, indicating that my time with him was over.

'Nothing else, Rob? You won't go wrong working for Douglas.'

I walked toward the door, and then, before leaving, I turned and asked,

'There is just one more question?'

'Yes?'

'I'm not sure if you know that I'm from interstate. So, where is Coldstream?'

'In the Yarra Valley.'

'Oh. And where is the Yarra Valley?'

'Northeast of Melbourne, about an hour's drive from here.'

I left Tony's office and stepped into the busy street. My career as a vet was beginning. At the kerb, I paused, drew in the city air, and felt Melbourne swallow me whole. I was lucky to land a job. But that wasn't the real reason I had taken the job with Doug. I'd met someone *special* in my second year a university, and the pull of that chance meeting was stronger than the need to return home, but I kept that to myself.

My parents had always imagined I'd return, and I knew that my decision would privately upset them.

And the someone *special person* never guessed my feelings for her, not until much later, when the tide of life had already turned for us both.

And in ways I could never have imagined, my choice to stay, to take the job with Doug, shaped everything that followed. Everything.

3 – SLEEPING IN THE DOG HOUSE

By my second day at the practice, I'd already been re-branded as 'Robbie'. Jimmy Dunne, who I later learnt was a longtime mate of my new boss, Dr Doug Campbell, strolled into the waiting room, leaned on the counter, and found me there.

I smiled and asked, 'Can I help you?'

'I'm Jimmy. Is Dougie in?'

'I'll check. Will he know what it's about?'

'Oh, yes. I come in every morning at about this time.'

I left and went out the back into the surgery prep room.

'There's a Jimmy out the front for you. He said you'd know what it's about.'

In response, Doug called out, 'Yes! Jimmy, come through.'

'So you're Dougie's new vet?' he said extending a hand in greeting and beaming a smile.

'Yes. I am. Good to meet you, Jimmy.'

Snippets of a Vet's Life

He was an older man, perhaps in his forties. He had a rugged face and a disorganised mop of light brown hair on his head. He was lean, wiry, and radiated energy, and, as I was to discover, always had some outlandish new project,

'Jimmy comes in most mornings, and we have a coffee break together, so you will see a lot of Jimmy,' Doug explained.

'So you're... Robbie,' and with that, I was rechristened forever in the practice.

Our clients always called me Rob, but to Jimmy and later Doug, I was always, from then on, 'Robbie.'

'Dougie tells me that you are from interstate, and this is your first job?'

'Yep. I guess you could say I'm newly minted. Are you a farmer, Jimmy?' He had that farmer look about him.

'A farmer! Well, yes, you could describe me as a farmer,' and they both laughed.

'Jimmy does lots of things...sails a boat, owns and runs the Coldstream Airfield, has a few cows, and so, yes, Jimmy is sort of a farmer,' Doug explained, and then asked, 'Who would like a cup of coffee?'

And so started a morning ritual that I came to cherish.

***

For the first few days, I drove back to the city each night and slept at a friend's house, and then back to the Yarra Valley for work the following morning. This arrangement was only a stopgap. I needed to figure out how to be in the Yarra Valley at night, especially when I was on duty, which was to start in the following week.

Towards the end of the first week, Doug raised the subject one morning while we were having coffee with Jimmy.

'So, Robbie. Have you given any thought to where you will live now?'

'Yes. Next week. When I start out-of-hours duty, I've been thinking that driving back and forth here each night and morning is not going to work.'

'You might be able to find something locally, like an apartment or even a house,' Jimmy added and then offered, 'I could help you with finding something. Robbie'

As I was to learn, Jimmy always helped people.

'In the meantime, Robbie, I have a spare camp stretcher, and we could put it in the kennel room until you find something better,' Doug offered.

Jimmy smiled and added, 'You aren't even married Robbie, and you're already sleeping in the dog house!'

That night, back in Melbourne, I gathered my few worldly possessions, including my precious lecture notes, and the following day, I left my university friends and their room to move to the country.

When I was at University, I lived at Trinity College, and in my day, we had maids who would make our beds, clean our study, and serve us dinner at night. They were called the maids, but they were not servants. But all that had changed, and I was now living in the back of the Coldstream Vet Clinic, sleeping on a camp stretcher, and not a maid in sight. Such is life.

For the next few weeks, the clinic dog room was my bedroom. Sometimes, a sick dog would stay overnight in a treatment cage in the room. Often, they would be quiet, but the occasional patient would not welcome being separated from its master and would howl or bark for most of the night. As much as I could do to console the distressed dog, it would continue to howl, and my dreaming would be interrupted.

After one particularly sleepless night, I attended to the morning in clinic cases while Doug made farm calls to his cattle clients. Towards lunchtime, I was working out back when I heard the clinic doorbell sound, indicating somebody's arrival.

She stood there in the waiting room, quiet, dignified, and wearing gloves.

'Hello,' I said and smiled at her.

'Is Dr Campbell in?' she said in a calm but commanding, slightly English voice. She had grey hair neatly swept back and was dressed in an English country style. She had a commanding presence merely by the way she stood.

'I'm afraid he is not. Was he expecting you?'

'No. But I have an injured dog. We were working with the cattle, and unfortunately, Skipper got kicked. Will Dr Campbell be long?'

'We expect him back shortly. But perhaps I can help you? I'm his new vet if you are in a hurry.'

'That's very good of you. If it is no trouble, perhaps I could leave Skipper with you. He's been here before, so his details are in my file.'

'OK. Yes, I'm happy to admit him, and what name would he be under....'

'Pamela Pridham,' and with that, she handed me Skipper's lead, turned and left.

As I was to learn, she was always a lady of few words and, at times, abrupt. However, she was not rude; she was just shy and sometimes sharp in her commands.

She turned back towards me, and directed, 'And could you ask Dr. Campbell to call me once he has seen Skipper?'

'Certainly...' and before I could continue, she was gone, leaving me with the injured dog.

About ten minutes later, Doug walked through the door. I was examining Skipper and told him about the situation.

'So, Robbie. You've met Pamela Pridham. She's only recently returned to Coldstream after spending most of her life overseas, mainly in England.'

'Right. I thought she had a slightly English air about her.'

'She does. She's back now, living in Emmerton House. That's the big one on the way out of town toward Yarra Glen. She can seem a little reserved, probably because she's shy, but she carries herself with that quiet authority that comes from her background. Not smug, just… steady.'

We both attended to Skipper's injuries, and while I held his collar, Doug injected a small quantity of local anaesthetic into the edge of a small gash on Skipper's chest.

While we waited for the drug to work, Doug asked, 'Robbie, have you made any advances on finding somewhere to live?'

'Getting there' was my response, but I had made limited progress. The central issue was that I needed to find a place that would eventually allow me to keep a horse.

Doug deftly stitched the edges of the wound together. After injecting Skipper with a long-acting antibiotic to stop any infection, I put him in a cage.

'I'll give the owner a ring, tell her that he is ready for discharge and to come back in 10 days for you to check the wound and take out the stitches. OK with you, Robbie?'

I thought no more at that time of Skipper and his slightly reserved owner.

4 – THE MATRON AND MR BROWN

Like a lamb to the slaughter, I was the fresh-faced new vet in town, always smiling, wearing a tie and ironed collar, and still unaware of the local power dynamics.

Samantha, the clinic nurse, handed me the phone with a slight raise of her eyebrows and a whispered warning.

'It's the Matron.'

Not just a matron. She was the Matron of the local Coldstream and District Community Hospital. I'd met her a few weeks earlier when she brought in her dog, a retired greyhound named Speedy (no irony intended) for his annual vaccination.

Most vet students of my generation carried a secret, oddly sentimental fondness for greyhounds. The ones who weren't quick enough on the track often ended up in anatomy labs as cadavers for second-year dissection. Something was unsettling about it at the time, though we rarely said so out loud. In real life, though, greyhounds are gentle, graceful, and oddly noble, and a pleasure to treat. But of course, I didn't tell the Matron about my connection to the breed.

At our first meeting, I examined Speedy and administered his annual vaccinations. Like most greyhounds, true to form, he was a joy to examine. He just stood stoically on the examination room table. He did not resist as I looked in his mouth and checked his heart, lungs, eyes, and ears.

While I checked her dog, the Matron chatted about many topics and people whom I did not know. She asked me many questions, some of which were slightly private. Did I have a girlfriend? How long had I been a vet? I answered as best I could. At times, I felt that I was being interviewed. She also mentioned that she had a daughter who was about the same age as me.

I patted Speedy under his jaw and asked, 'Anything else?'

'No. You have done a thorough job. Thank you.'

As she was about to leave, there was a final question. 'Do you like opera?'

I thought the question was unusual, but I answered that I did and explained that I had attended a few when I was a student living in Trinity College.

'That's good, Rob. Thanks. I'll be in touch,' but her parting words, about the opera, left me wondering.

Later that day, Doug received a telephone call from her, and after he put down the receiver, said,

Snippets of a Vet's Life

'So, Robbie, you've met the Matron. She liked you. Well done. She'll spread the word. She's good for business. They'll all be 'twittering' about you around town now,' and I saw that he had a slight glint in his eyes.

I looked at him, not entirely understanding what 'a twitter' meant, but I smiled back.

And now, a few weeks later, she was on the phone, asking for me.

'Good morning, Matron. How can I help you?'

During our first meeting, I quickly formed the impression that the Matron was a force to be reckoned with, and now, during this phone call, I was to gather more evidence in support.

'Has a Mr. Brown made a time to see you?'

Without waiting for an answer, she continued, 'Because if he hasn't, he will. I have told him to see you. He's a day patient at the hospital and worried about his dog. It's got a lump. And. . .'

This phone call occurred about three weeks into my career as a Vet.

I was officially the 'New Vet' or the 'Young Vet.'

Being newly graduated, I was still coming to terms with some of the subtleties of being a vet and a professional, so while the Matron was talking, I was considering how to answer her question:

'Has Mr. Brown made an appointment?'

Was this information considered confidential? Did her position as the respected Matron of the local hospital elevate her into 'somebody who could be told?' The Matron was contacting me for what, as she went on to explain, seemed to be a good reason: Mr. Brown had only weeks to live. Clearly, the Matron considered me someone with whom she could share this bit of confidential information.

'So, Rob, as I was saying, when he comes in, if the lump is bad, DON'T TELL HIM! He only lives for the dog. OK? Bye'

Click.

She was gone, and I was left with a problem. However, this was not the first time I had encountered this situation. A few years earlier, when I was a vet student, I received the unsettling news that my grandmother had been unwell for a while and one day, she collapsed and was admitted to the hospital.

My father called me, and the decision was made that I would travel from Melbourne to home on the overnight train. The next morning, he collected me from the station and drove me to the hospital.

We both stood silently in the lift. My father was very close to his mother, and I realised that this was a stressful time for him. We walked towards her room, and as I was about to enter, he stopped me and said,

'She hasn't got long to go, son. She's got liver cancer, but to save her the worry, we have told her that she is getting better. Don't tell her if she asks,' and with that, gently pushed me into her room, alone.

She was jaundiced and looked tired but pleased to see me, and I could see that in her eyes, she was 'weary of the world.'

I sat alongside, on her bed, and she pulled herself up, looking deep into me, and asked,

'Am I dying?'

As she looked at me, with her question still in the air, I chose to ignore my father's well-intentioned direction, and answered my Granny with the single word,

'Yes.'

She took my hand, squeezed it, relaxed her face, and, looking at me, gently said,

'Thank you.'

We talked, and talked as never before, about 'life' until she was worn out, and then it was time to go. As she closed her eyes, I quietly left.

It was the last time I saw her. She died when I was on the train back to Melbourne, and my other life. My father never knew that I had told the truth to his mother. I have always felt that I did the right thing by my grandmother and my father.

And now, the Matron was seeking a similar untruth, for a similar reason.

I greeted Mr Brown as he entered the examination room.

'Hello. I'm Rob. How can I help you?'

I helped him lift a West Highland Terrier onto the examination table. Mr. Brown was very thin and frail, and his breathing was laboured. There was a slight blue tinge to his lips, and the effort of lifting Jock onto the table had exhausted him. He sat down in the examination room chair, out of breath. I waited, and after a while, he regained his strength and said, 'I'm worried about Jock. He's lost some weight lately, and I have found a lump in his groin.'

I felt the lump, as he, with some respiratory effort, continued, 'I asked the Matron what she thought, and she said it was probably nothing…but I'm worried. It is nothing, isn't it?'

'Let's check him out fully,' I said as I started to examine him.

The lump was about 2 cm in diameter and was high up on the inside of Jock's left hind leg. It was possibly an enlarged lymph node. I was suspicious. I felt other lymph nodes. They were also enlarged, but not as much as the lump Mr. Brown had discovered. Jock's anal temperature was normal.

Snippets of a Vet's Life

Without further testing, a reasonable diagnosis was that Jock had lymphoma, and in the mid '70s, not a lot could be done to cure the condition. Jock was unlikely to be alive in six months. And the Matron's admonition was still ringing in my ears, 'Mr. Brown is dying, and he is only living for his dog!'

His face portrayed a hopeful look as he asked,

'What do you think?'

'Well,' I said, deflecting his question, 'I can see why you are a bit worried. How long has the lump been there?'

'Not long. I'm sure it wasn't there until recently,' and this added to my unsaid presumptive diagnosis of lymphoma, which is a malignant disease of the lymph system that can present quickly in some cases.

And then he asked the question I was dreading.

'Jock's going to be OK, isn't he?'

I thought of my grandmother, and the Matron stern command. I did my best to have a comforting smile.

'Yes, Mr Brown. I think Jock will be fine. I will give you some tablets to give him every day, and if you follow the directions, Jock will start to put on weight again, and the lump will get smaller. He might also drink more water.'

'What caused the lump?'

'Oh. It's nothing. I feel them all the time. I'm not worried about it. It's just something that old dogs can get.'

I felt terrible, but it had the desired effect. His face lit up, and I could see I had given a welcome answer. I handed him the dose of cortisone tablets and wrote the directions by hand.

'Can you read my writing, Mr. Brown?'

He put on his glasses and read the handwritten drug label.

'Yes, I can. Prednisolone. Is that like cortisone? I think that I'm taking the same drug. I haven't got long… I have lung cancer. And now Jock is taking the same medication…' He had a questioning look.

'I'm sorry to hear that, Mr. Brown, about your lungs. But cortisone has a variety of uses. I think Jock is going to be fine.'

It was a lie, but it had the desired effect. Mr. Brown looked happy again, and after I lifted Jock off the table, he got out of the chair, and stood up. I handed him the lead, and they both left. I did not see Mr. Brown or Jock again, but I was left with an unanswerable question:

Did I do 'right' by doing 'good'?

As a vet, I had a licence to use death as a treatment, but did that give me a licence to also kill hope?

5 – UP CLOSE AND PERSONAL WITH A MARE

Doug put the phone down.

'Well, Robbie. How would you feel about pregnancy testing a mare?'

I had been a working vet for a few days, mainly conducting simple consultations, including one with a dog experiencing diarrhoea and another with a cat sneezing excessively. I also did a few annual checkups before administering the yearly vaccinations to several dogs and a cat. There was also a rabbit with a eye discharge.

Nothing too taxing and within my capabilities as a new graduate.

But pregnancy testing a mare, which involved standing behind and inserting my lubricated arm into a mare's rectum to palpate her uterus, would be extending me, and I would be attending the owner's property alone without my boss being available in the background.

Before I left on my first out call, Doug advised, 'Now. You will need lube, and luckily, they have a horse crush, so you will be fine standing behind the mare. I have spoken to Jane and Sonia. They own the mare and are happy you are doing the pregnancy test instead of me. Let me show you where they are on the map. Centre Road, Parslow's Bridge.'

About half an hour later, I arrived. The trip had taken me past a few small vineyards, many small farms, a cow or two grazing near the side of the road, and a few horses. People were dotted here and there, in fields or walking alongside the road, going about their daily tasks, and one or two waved to me as I passed them. I was beginning to realise that it was a friendly community. I was in a good place.

I was greeted by two middle-aged women, Jane and Sonia. One of them said, as she turned and walked away,

'Come this way. We have the mare in the yard waiting for you.'

As I was to learn, Jane was always in a hurry, always doing something, and would sometimes lose her cool and get angry. Sonia was the complete opposite. Nothing seemed to upset her calm countenance. She always moved unhurriedly and was never flustered, even when being berated by her friend. I ran to catch up with retreating Jane.

Snippets of a Vet's Life

'So Doug tells us that this is the first time you have preg-tested a mare,' Jane said.

'Well. No... that is not strictly correct. I have practised on a few mares during the last year of my course. But it is the first time since I graduated.'

'All I ask is that you be careful and not tear her. I believe in giving you new guys a go,' she said, adding to my psychological burden.

Jane was referring to the risk that during the procedure, which involved the vet introducing an arm into a mare's rectum, part of the rectal wall could tear, and the mare would then be at a real risk of suffering peritonitis and probably dying as a result.

'I will be. But, there is always a risk...'

'If you're not sure, then don't do it, and we'll wait for Doug,' was her response.

'I'm sure, ' I said as I patted the mare on her rump, hoping I sounded confident.

But inwardly, I was anything but confident. I knew how easily I could damage the mare if I were not sufficiently careful.

'What's her name?' I asked to lighten the mood.

'Dorothy. One of my favourites. She may not be in foal, but I was expecting her to come in season recently, and she didn't. So I'm wondering if somehow my little stallion...? There was a storm a few weeks ago, and he broke through the fence during the night. I found them together in the morning, and as we all know, boys will be boys!'

And to add to my stress, Dorothy was one of Jane's favourites. Great.

'Was she in season at the time?' I asked as though nothing was troubling me.

'I didn't think so, but…maybe. Let's find out.'

We walked towards the mare, who stood silently in a crush that comfortably restrained her.

The weather was unusually warm, and I was grateful we were under a tree and there was a slight breeze. Alongside the crush was a bucket of water. I wore a tie, so I tucked the end into the top of my shirt, rolled up my right sleeve, washed my arm, and applied some lube directly to my right arm. This was before the availability of inexpensive shoulder-length arm protecting gloves, so it was skin-to-rectum time.

I walked towards the mare's rear end. A low gate prevented the mare from backing out and, in theory, prevented her from kicking out backwards. Standing behind her, and side on, I lifted her tail and gently introduced my right index finger into her rectum. There was some resistance, but I waited. Once the mare had relaxed her anus, my first finger was followed by a second, and again, after waiting for her to relax, a third, then all of my right hand, and with a plop, my hand was in her rectum.

Snippets of a Vet's Life

I paused, with my right foot forward and my body turned to the left, and with my left foot behind, for support, I was able to push my right hand gently, and then my arm, further into her insides, gently along her rectum. As I progressed, her rectum clamped onto my arm. I waited for her to relax at each slight move I made, and then proceeded. I was being very cautious, and the mare was moving about a bit. I waited and then pushed a bit further, feeling all the time for her uterus below the rectal wall. She shifted again as I used the wall of the rectum as a glove and felt around inside her abdomen for her womb.

And there it was. Below my fingers: her uterus.

Gently, I moved my hand from the centre of the uterus, first to the left and then to the right. The mare shifted. I waited. She relaxed. I continued palpating her uterus. And then I felt what I was searching for: a swelling in the right horn of her uterus. She was pregnant!

This was my first positive pregnancy test in a mare. She was much more along than the standard 28 day manual pregnancy test, but it was my first time alone. I was elated.

As I was about to announce the result, I felt the mare's rump tense very slightly, and with slight movement forward and her head going down, she explosively kicked both hind legs behind her, and simultaneously, my arm was expelled. It happened so quickly. She then stood calmly again, as though nothing had happened, and I picked myself up off the ground behind the crush. She had 'double-barrelled' me in response to me perhaps putting too much pressure on her uterus. As part of good practice, I had learnt during training, was to always position myself side-on behind a mare, just in case she should try to kick me in response to whatever I was doing at her rear end.

The mare had kicked out in the direction of my head, but because I was positioned sideways to her, her hooves went on either side of me, and my head remained intact as I fell to the ground.

Swallowing my real reaction, absolute fear, I mustered as much sangfroid as I could gather. 'Well. That was lucky,' I muttered. 'It can happen. Part of the job. No really, I'm fine.'

Both women attempted to assist me in getting up while apologising for the mare's behaviour. As before, as if I was not worried, I nervously repeated, 'Well, it can happen. It's part of the job. I'm fine.'

They both looked at me, and Jane, laughing, said, 'Well. I don't know how you feel, Rob, but you have gone completely white in the face!'

'Really? Anyway, she's pregnant, which is good news.'

They continued to smile as I cleaned my arm, removed my tie, and made to leave.

Snippets of a Vet's Life

'Anything else that I can do for you?' I asked.

As I left, I considered how close I had come to being knocked out by the mare. 'Lucky me,' I thought, and for the first time, I realised that my dream job, being one day an equine veterinarian, involved risks not experienced by other members of my profession.

It could be, at times, perilous. And it was a job that could kill me.

Rod Graham

6 – THE GOAT

Before the advent of mobile phones, being 'on duty' as a vet significantly constrained the freedom to do your own thing.

The vet on call always had to be reachable, which usually meant that if they were in a relationship, their partner would take calls and pass on messages. If the vet, as in my case, lived at the clinic, there was an expectation that the vet would answer all phone calls, including essential and non-essential ones, such as, 'When is the clinic next open..?' or 'I want to make a time for the vet to pregnancy test my cows' and so forth. I wasn't lamenting this role; it was just part of the job.

On Saturday evening, my first weekend on duty, I turned on the clinic's answering machine, left a message stating that I would be back by a particular time, and went to a local restaurant for a quick dinner and the comfort of a book.

The answer machine was blinking red on my return, and my heart rate slightly increased.

Snippets of a Vet's Life

'Hi,' a female voice said. 'Is that the new vet? I've heard a lot about you from my friend, and I think my goat is feeling a bit unwell. Could you give me a call? I think you need to see him tonight,' and she left a contact number.

Her name was Helen. Over the phone, she couldn't give me a clear picture of what was wrong with her goat, but I told her I would be there within half an hour.

The street numbering wasn't what it should have been, and initially, I had knocked on the wrong door. This was my first experience with after hours home visits and was to be the start of many years of frustration in finding where clients actually lived, e.g. finding the white house that had no fence, no street number, and was at the end of the street instead of where they thought they lived, 'No 42, and you can't miss it'.

I knocked. I waited. I knocked again. No response. Nobody home? Was it the wrong house again? I began to feel a slight panic, fearing that I would be late. Perhaps, I had have written the house number down incorrectly?

As I turned away, I heard a quiet voice say, from the other side of the closed door,

'Is that the vet?'

I returned to the closed door.

'Yes. Hi. I'm Rob the vet, ' I said, adding, to give her confidence, 'We spoke on the phone. Is that Helen?'

The door opened slightly, and a woman in her forties popped her head out. I smiled in greeting, but she initially looked past me and towards the road. She looked worried, but then, seemingly satisfied that nobody else was behind me, she smiled at me.

'Hi, yes. I'm Helen. Thanks for coming. '

She then fully opened the door and gestured for me to go inside. Once inside, she quickly closed the door.

'I'm sorry about that. But I have to be careful. My ex-husband...,' but she didn't finish the sentence.

'Sit down...Rob? I'm just about to have a coffee. Would you like one?

'Yes. I'm Rob. Thanks. Coffee would be great,' and she left. I looked around the room. I noticed there were many photographs of the woman. There were pictures of her as a teenager, as a young woman, and more recent photos. There were no photos of a man and his wife.

I waited.

There was a clock on the wall, and it had a loud tick. 8:10 pm. I wondered when I would return to the clinic and what else awaited me on the answering machine. I waited. The room was cluttered, and the remains of a recent meal were scattered on a small table. Perhaps she had been watching television while waiting for me?

I wondered where she kept her sick goat. Perhaps in the backyard? I listened. I heard a distant door open and then close. I picked up a book from the coffee table and flicked through it. I put the book down and stood up as Helen re-entered the room, holding a tray.

'Oh, how very polite you are. Please sit down. Hope you don't mind, but I just had to get out of those other clothes into something fresh.' I thought this was odd at the time, but that was all.

For all my formal education, I was not that street-smart, and I knew nothing about the opposite sex.

I was the youngest of three brothers, attended an all-boys agricultural school and lived a relatively sheltered childhood in many ways.

Amanda Brussel was an honest 'English rose', and I became enamoured of her. She lived across the road from where I lived as a kid. Some days we would play outside like any normal young children.

Gradually, we both grew older, and one day, I saw her in a *different light*.

I became slightly embarrassed in her presence, and she seemed to know much more about *things* than I did.

Secretly, I fell in love for the first time.

And then, a year or two later, there was Claire McAdams. I met her while horse riding and fell in love for the second time. I dreamed and planned a life together, but then one day she introduced me to Nick, her boyfriend.

I had spent weeks preparing to ask her to a school dance, and I was about to pop the question when the boyfriend surfaced. I had put an extra heavy spray of underarm deodorant on that day, but Nick's appearance dashed my hopes of a future life with the secretly adored Claire.

Even at University, I had little success with the opposite gender.

Jackie caught my attention during Orientation week. From then on, I spent many weeks sitting as close as possible to her in lectures. Some days, I even got to sit next to her. I was always planning my next move. Girls don't understand how much time a boy spends planning his *next move*.

Finally, the big day.

She was studying in the Botany library of the Biology Building upstairs. I entered the room and saw her. She smiled at me. Was it a *special* smile, I wondered. Was that a sign? Or was she just being polite? I was unsure, but I was determined to ask her out. I had lost a lot of sleep thinking about Jackie. I was worried because I had noticed that Warwick, a second-year vet student, had recently engaged with her at lunchtime. Was Warwick trying to move in on my territory? This is how young men think. Or so I thought. And Warwick seemed to have it all. Most of all, he was confident, and I wasn't.

Snippets of a Vet's Life

I approached her table. She looked up and smiled. Was that a 'Yes, I'm thrilled to see you smile', or merely a, 'Hi Rob. What do you want, smile?' I wondered.

'Hi, Jackie,' I blurted out without waiting for her to answer. 'Would you like to go to a film this weekend? With me?'

'Oh, you are so nice. But I can't, Rob. I'm going away with my boyfriend.'

Boyfriend! I was shattered. Another one. Just like Claire McAdams. Did every girl have a boyfriend? When would I be introduced one day as somebody's boyfriend?

'OK,' I said, smiling awkwardly. 'Perhaps another time?'

'Yes. Perhaps,' she said. I retreated to my seat and my books. Soon she got up and left the library. 'See you at the next lecture,' she said as she went. And I felt stupid, embarrassed, hurt, and mostly disappointed. I didn't go to the lecture.

'How do you take your coffee?' Helen, the goat owner, asked, interrupting my thoughts.

'Black. No sugar,' I replied.

'So do I,' she said, 'Isn't that amazing?' and sat down next to me on the couch as she poured. 'I see that you've been looking at my books,' and she leaned forward and straightened the books on the coffee table. 'Are you interested in fashion?' Without waiting for my answer, she continued, 'I used to be a fashion model.'

'Were you?' I said, attempting to be polite.

'Yes. Would you like to see some of my pictures from my modelling days?'

'Yes,' I said again, being polite.

She left the room and, after a few minutes, returned holding a large folio. She sat next to me again and opened the book, resting it on both our knees. I hadn't noticed before, but I now smelled perfume. Yes. It was definitely perfume.

I began to feel a bit uncomfortable, and my thoughts turned to the goat. My discomfort grew when, after reaching over to turn a page in her folio book, her knee brushed against mine.

I looked at the clock. It was now 9:30 pm.

She continued turning the pages, giving me a visual tour of her life. And even though I moved slightly away, our knees kept touching each other. I remained polite and feigned interest. I also felt a bit hot on my face. Was I blushing? Finally, we arrived at the last page. It was a wedding photo.

'Is that your husband?' Again, I was polite, but secretly, I wondered about her sick goat. Where was the goat?

'Yes. That's him. He's a piece of....,' and I formed the distinct impression that she didn't like him anymore.

Snippets of a Vet's Life

'That's been really interesting, Helen. Now, perhaps if you could show me where your goat is?'

'Don't worry. The goat's out the back. I can't tell you how hard the last few weeks have been. Oh. I'm so rude. I'll get you another coffee, or perhaps, something stronger?'

'Coffee's fine. I don't drink.'

And then she spent the next hour relaying how difficult her marriage had been, with me making appropriate enquiries, asking pertinent questions, and acting interested.

But I wasn't. I was just polite. And the goat?

When I was young, I was so very, very…polite. I wore a tie and ensured my shirts were clean and freshly ironed. I now realise that in many ways, I was socially inept.

It was now 10:15 pm.

'Well, that has been very interesting. I'm sorry that you have had such a tough time. Um…' and I stood up. 'It's getting late; perhaps now may be a good time to look at your goat,' I said.

'That's OK. I checked him before, when I went out for the second coffee. He's better. Actually, he appeared better before you arrived, but I didn't want to disappoint you. And we seemed to be having a good time together, just chatting. And you have been so interested.'

I wasn't sure why she thought I would be disappointed that her goat was now better. Had she told me when I had arrived, I could have left and had an early night. Sometimes, people think differently from me, and this was one of those times. I was starting to feel uncomfortable again.

'Well, I'd better be off now,' I said, unsure of what was happening.

'Oh. Don't go! Meeting you is so much fun. And I like you…' But I picked up my bag and went to the front door. 'Would you like a drink before you go? '

'No, thanks. I don't drink,' I reiterated. I was now feeling very uncomfortable with the whole situation.

'Is there a charge?' she asked, with her head tilted to one side and brushing hair out of one eye.

'Interesting. There should be, but since I didn't do anything, with your goat being better, I don't know…' I paused to consider her question further and concluded, 'No. Since your goat is OK, I don't think I can charge you.'

'You're so sweet,' and with that, leaned towards me and kissed me on my cheek.

I was shocked and stumbled back out the door, dropping my bag as I went. 'I really must go.'

'Are you sure you don't want a drink? Another coffee? Or something…' Her head was strangely on one side, and she looked slightly upwards at me. I also noted that she was now playing with her hair.

'No. I'm OK. Thanks for offering, but I've had enough coffee.'

'Perhaps a soda water?' And she put her hand on my arm.

'No, I'm good. I've got to get going,' I turned towards my car. Over my shoulder, still being ever so polite, I said, 'Helen, it's been great meeting you. Bye, and good luck!'

And I left.

The following Monday morning, Doug asked about my first weekend on duty.

'So you met a lady and her…goat?' He had a wry smile on his face.

'Yes, Helen, but not the goat,' I replied. 'So, to tell the truth, because I didn't actually do anything, I didn't charge her for the call. I was a bit unsure how to handle the situation…' but before I could finish, he interrupted me.

'Next time, Robbie, always make sure you charge if you are called out. Even if you don't have to do anything. You charge for your time. OK?'

'OK,' but I was uncomfortable.

Rod Graham

Looking back, the signs were all there, and any good detective would have seen them, but I was still learning: I was the goat.

Snippets of a Vet's Life

7 – THE GREEN COTTAGE

Jimmy was in attendance, as was his habit, for morning coffee, a week after I started working at the Coldstream Vet Clinic. The topic of my accommodation came up again.

'So, Robbie. Have you found anywhere to live yet?' Jimmy asked.

To this day, I do not understand why I did not rent a flat in Coldstream, except that I suspect I was probably short of funds, as many graduating vets are. I suffered another sleepless night because I once again shared the dog room with a complaining dog staying with us post-surgery. Therefore, I found Jimmy's question relevant.

This time, my roommate was Carl, a male Visla dog, who spent much of the night restless and whining. He was still feeling the effects of the intravenous anaesthetic, and I imagined that he was in discomfort post-abdominal surgery. Initially, I felt compassion for him, but about 3:00 a.m., that feeling was gradually replaced by annoyance at the constant interruption to my sleep on the camp stretcher.

So Jimmy's question was by chance right on target.

'No. Not yet. But the other day, when I was driving back from Healesville, I saw what looked to be a derelict weatherboard house next to a set of big green gates. It looked to be part of the Emmerton House Estate.'

'Yes, I know it. That's the old gardener's cottage, but nobody has lived there for years. So, are you thinking of living there?'

'Well. It did occur to me that it might be suitable, if I could only find out who was in charge of it. Who do I call?'

'Ring Pammy Pridham. She will be the person to ask since she moved into the main house a few years ago.'

I remembered that I had met her recently when she had brought her injured dog, Skipper, in for attention.

'You sure? She won't mind?' 'No, Pammy is fine. She's reserved, but she's a good stick. I've known her since I was a child. She grew up around here before she went to England and married. Her husband died some years ago, and she eventually came back home. She's been on her own since then, but she knows everyone and carries herself with quiet authority.'

Later that day, I looked up her client card and called. It was to be the first of only two telephone conversations I had with her.

The second, and last, was near the end of my tenure in the Green Cottage. I had returned from tending to a horse with colic, and I went to turn into my parking spot outside the set of big green gates that guarded the exit of her property.

A van blocked me. On its side was the logo of a local television station, Channel Nine.

There was a recent anniversary of the 'Wave Hill Walk Off', where, in August 1966, a strike by Indigenous workers for better working conditions was considered a significant influence on Aboriginal land rights in Australia. An English pastoral company owned Wave Hill Station at the time, which is why the TV station was interested in Mrs Pridham. She was a member by marriage of the family.

I parked, got out, and looked through the slats in the green wooden gates.

Inside was a small group of men, one of whom was holding a camera facing towards the big house in the distance. Towards her home. The men should not have been inside the gates. With good lenses, they could look into her house, her home, and…her refuge. I went inside and called.

'Yes?', she said, with her quiet, hesitant voice.

'I apologise for calling, Mrs Pridham, but you should know that a television camera is aimed at the back of your house. They are from Sixty Minutes on Channel Nine.'

'Oh, no!' I could hear a brief intake of air. 'Thank you, Dr McBride.'

A 'click' ended what was our last telephone call.

The first phone call I made was not long after Jimmy had told me, over our morning coffee, to give her a call.

'Pamela Pridham' was the short answer.

'Hi, Mrs Pridham. Rob McBride here. I met you at the Vet Clinic the other day when you brought Skipper in to be stitched. I'm Doug's new vet.

'Hello. Yes, I remember you.'

'How's Skipper?' seemed a good place to start, but she cut short my small talk with an abrupt response.

'OK... Is that all?'

The suddenness of her response took me aback. Her manner indicated: get to the point.

'Mrs Pridham, I won't take much more of your time, but I am calling to ask if I could rent the old cottage on Healesville Road.'

'Cottage?'

I suddenly thought that perhaps Jimmy's information had been incorrect, and that the cottage had no connection to her. But, as it turned out, he was correct.

'Yes. The one with the green roof, next to the big green gates, and on the...'

She interrupted before I could continue.

Snippets of a Vet's Life

'You mean the Green Cottage,' said as a statement, not a question.

'Probably. It's just that I'm sleeping...'

And before I could continue, she answered with an emphatic 'No'.

I have learnt never to accept 'no' as a negative, but merely as the start of a conversation.

'No? That's a pity. I'm currently sleeping in the dog room at the vet clinic on a camp stretcher, and I'm looking for somewhere, if only for a short term. And I was hoping that perhaps, maybe...?'

'No.' She repeated, this time not as sternly. I heard what I perceived to be a slight movement in her position, and so I continued.

'I plan to keep a horse, and my problem is that I need somewhere with a few acres.'

'A horse?'

'Yes,' I said, fearing this added need may have ended my chances.

But it had a reverse effect. She seemed suddenly to warm to me, and we spoke for a few more minutes, mostly about my equestrian activities, and finally, she said,

'If you like, Dr. McBride, I could meet you at the cottage next Tuesday and show you why I can't rent it to you, or for that matter, anybody. Goodbye.'

Rod Graham

Click.

I could be late at times, but my appointment with Mrs Pridham at the Green Cottage was at 10:00 am, and I was on time, right on the hour.

After having breakfast at the local Coldstream Road House, I drove out of Coldstream towards the big house that guarded the intersection of the Yarra Glen and Healesville roads. I took the right fork towards Healesville, following the long sweep of the highway that formed the boundary of her estate. About 400 metres along the road, on the left, was the Green Cottage, and Mrs Pridham was standing at the front gate. I parked and greeted her. She politely responded as she opened the garden gate.

The loose wire gate protested loudly as it scraped across the path. Nearly 50 years later, I can still hear the sound. I can't forget, either, the noise of the key in the back door. A clunk, followed by a rattle and then a heave-ho to the door as it opened. I followed her in.

'Well, Dr McBride,' she said (and as I came to experience, she always referred to me by my formal name, except once). This is why I'm unable to rent the cottage to you. It is derelict, and nobody has lived in this cottage for many years.'

We stood in the kitchen, and I could see the adjacent paddocks through the two opposite windows. To the left of the fireplace was an obvious hole in the wooden floor. It was about the size of a large saucepan, and underneath, about a metre deep, I could see the underlying soil. A doorway was to the right of the ancient wood-burning black metal oven in a brick fireplace.

'You can try that, but I don't think the door has been opened for years. It is the entrance to the sitting room.'

I tried the handle. It turned, but time and the collapse of the foundations had distorted the frame, and I could not open the door. It was firmly wedged shut. I wouldn't gain entry to the sitting room for another few weeks, and only after I had used a car jack to raise the house onto new foundations.

'This is perfect," I said.

She looked surprised.

I explained, 'It is much better than the dog kennel room at the clinic, where I am currently sleeping.'

She went silent for a while and then said, 'Well, I guess you could stay here if you think it is right for you. I think it's uninhabitable, but I could see how it might work if you wish. But there are two requirements, Dr. McBride, that I want you to follow. That, in fact, you MUST follow.'

'Yes?'

'The first is that you respect my privacy, and the second is that you never ring me. If you need to contact me, please write me a letter and leave it at the post office in Coldstream. Is that possible?'

'Letter? Yes, I can do that. Thank you. I am sure you will have no trouble with me.'

'Didn't you say that you want to keep a horse?', pointing out the far kitchen window, 'You can use that five acre paddock next door.'

'When do you wish to move in?'

'Would today be too soon?'

She handed me the key, and that night, I exchanged sleeping in the clinic dog room for sleeping on the floor in the kitchen of the derelict Green Cottage.

When I arrived at work the following day, there was an envelope with my name handwritten on the front.

It was the first of many letters that crossed from her to me, and me to her.

'Dear Dr McBride, I have checked with my lawyer, who informed me that, for legal reasons, I am required to charge you rent. To that end, would asking for a peppercorn a year be too much? Pamela Pridham.'

What luck, I thought. She had given me a great gift. I could permanently move out of the dog room at the vet clinic and into my own accommodation. And I could keep a horse in the paddock next door.

And all for the cost of a peppercorn a year.

It was only years later that I realised how much this arrangement was to 'cost' me.

Snippets of a Vet's Life

There was no need for me to save, and then buy somewhere to live.

Sometimes, there is nothing so costly as something that is *free*.

8 – THE MATRON'S GIFT

About two weeks later, when I arrived at work, I greeted Doug and nodded towards Samantha, who was on the phone. She was Doug's nurse (whom I came to experience never warmed to me, probably because I had in some ways taken over some of her roles).

She put her hand over the receiver and, directing herself to Doug, said, 'The Matron is on the phone. She wants you to go to her property in Parslow's Bridge and drench her two horses. And today, if possible. It's her day off.'

He looked over at me. I knew Doug disliked dealing with horses, so it was no surprise when he said, 'Robbie. Want a trip to Parslow's Bridge before lunch?'

'Sure.' I was secretly a bit cautious of the Matron after she had put me in a difficult professional position with one of her patients, Mr Brown and his dog, not long after I had started work. Doug indicated to Samantha to hand him the phone.

'Morning, Matron. I have a lot booked today. How would you feel if I sent Robbie out to see you?'

Snippets of a Vet's Life

After the call had finished, he said, 'OK, Robbie. She's expecting you at 11.00 am to drench her horses. I assume that you've done that before.'

'Yes. I have. Won't be a problem,' I replied, full of confidence. One skill I was confident in was handling horses. I still thank my father for that.

In his day, he had been a Mounted Policeman in the Police Force until, while out riding one Saturday, he suffered a fall, causing a nasty head injury.

As my mother would tell me one day after they had separated, 'He became a changed man after the fall.'

After the accident, he suffered a lot from headaches and would retire to the seclusion of his bedroom. When he was having 'one of his headaches,' the house would necessarily become quiet.

He could also become angry in situations where the ferocity of his anger was not warranted.

I think he knew his angry outbursts were wrong, and instead of outbursts, he would get a tortured look on his face as he attempted to control his anger. It was not a time when men could openly admit to needing help, so he and his family suffered. There were good times and not-so-good times.

And, I was not surprised, on reflection, when I did seek help, that, at a young age, I also began to suffer from headaches and inward rages. I was not very good at expressing emotion. I had to learn this skill a long time after becoming an adult.

After the horse injury, he had to leave the Police Force, but he maintained his affection for horses. We always had a pony and later a racehorse, stabled in yards at the back of our house. The horses were the source of ongoing tension within the family, which was split between my father, my older brother, and me on one side and my mother and my other brother on the other.

Years later, after my parents had separated, my mother told me, 'If it wasn't for me working, you boys would not have had as much as you did.' Not that we had much. But I had a pony as a kid, and I am always thankful to my parents. And for this reason, I was comfortable handling horses.

Doug gave me directions to the Matron's property, and after packing my car, I backed out onto the highway and leisurely made my way to Parslow's Bridge.

On the way, I passed a few small orchards and a piggery. The road was not very busy, and once again, I felt happy with the job I had landed. A T-intersection on the road, featuring a small store and outside a single petrol bowser, along with two or three small houses, made up the beautifully named Parslow's Bridge. I turned left and, about 1 km further along the road, saw a sign on a metal gate, 'Tumble Wood'.

Snippets of a Vet's Life

The gate had fallen off its hinge and was tied to a post with some wire. I untwisted the wire, dragged the gate open, drove in, and started to shut it once again.

'There's no need to close it,' she called out from a slight hill a short distance from the gate. 'The horses are in the yard, and there is nothing else to get out. The cows have gone.'

So, I dropped the heavy gate, drove up the rise, and stopped outside the yards.

'Good morning, Matron,' for that is what most people called her. I only ever heard Jimmy and Doug refer to her by her first name.

She smiled at me. She had a generous smile. It was always welcoming. When I first met her, she was in her mid-forties with an attractive vibrancy. She was easy to be with and talked a lot, always with enthusiasm, but as I was to learn, I needed to keep my wits about me in dealing with her.

'So, Matron. Doug sent me to drench your horses.'

'I thought he would. He's been out here before to drench them, and I sensed that it isn't one of his favourite pastimes. I used to have cattle, and I think he preferred dealing with them.'

'No, he's fine with horses,' I said in support of my boss, 'But he knows that I have a special interest.'

I moved to the back of my car and removed a yellow plastic bucket and a red rubber stomach tube. I also retrieved a container full of Thiabendazole, a drug in powder form, which, when mixed with water, was administered through a nasogastric tube into a horse's stomach. This drug kills the common intestinal worms that infect many horses. The process of administering the powder mixed with water was called 'drenching' or 'worming' a horse. For the best management of horse intestinal worms, it was done about every 12 weeks.

As I got everything ready, I checked with the Matron and discovered that Doug had last drenched the Matron's horses about five months ago, so they were slightly overdue, as I reminded her.

'Yes, I know, but I thought I'd stretch it out a bit...to save on the cost of Doug coming out.'

'OK. I understand that, but for best results, every three months is recommended because of the worm cycle, before the worm larvae grow into adults and start producing eggs and larvae that can infect the pasture,' I said somewhat officiously, almost as though I had an unconscious need to impress her with my veterinary knowledge.

'There's no need for the lecture, Rob. I'm off the land, so I know about parasitic worms and worms in general. To be honest, the real reason I've waited is because last time, when Doug drenched them, one of the horses had a bloody nose after the tube came out, and the whole episode was a bit traumatic...for me and Doug,' and she flashed her smile, as if to indicate no malice in what she reported.

I tried to sound sympathetic and said something like, 'It can happen to the best of vets, but I trust it won't happen today.'

Maybe I was overly confident as I approached the first horse, a brown mare of medium height called Misty. She was tied to the yard's top rail by a lead rope and stood calmly as I untied the rope. I took the rubber tube out of the bucket of water and handed the Matron the pannikin holding the drench mixture.

I placed the end of the tube gently at the entrance of her left nostril, and then, with my fingers controlling her head by holding onto her muzzle, I deftly pushed the tube with my other hand up and into her nose. I stopped when I felt it slightly drop and hit the back of her throat. I waited, and as expected, the mare swallowed, and I continued pushing the tube into the nose, passing her throat, over her trachea, and into the oesophagus or gullet.

To ensure I was in the correct position, I put the other end of the tube in my mouth, blew, and saw a bubble of air travel down under the skin of her left neck, into her oesophagus. I was indeed in the correct position: I was in her gullet and not in her windpipe or trachea. I further checked by pulling the tube out of her nose for a few centimetres and then back in, and I could see it under the skin rising up, then going down her neck in the gullet as it ran down the left side of her neck.

'OK,' I said, attaching a plastic funnel to the exterior end of the tube at the same time. 'We are in. Can you pour the drench into the funnel for me now?'

And she did. Once the funnel was full of the drug/water mixture, I raised it above my head, and under gravity, it flowed into the mare. With a quick hand motion, I removed the tube, making sure it slid out gently. Sometimes, if the tube is removed too quickly, the inner end can flip up as it leaves the throat and hits the inner, highly vascular lining of the inside of the horse's nose.

But not this time. Success!

'That went well. Rob. You are so calm.'

'Thanks. I have an admission to make, Matron. Even though I have done this procedure many times as a student, Misty is the first horse I have stomach-drenched as a qualified vet.'

'That's an achievement that should be celebrated.'

But her other horse was not as compliant as Misty had been. Pablo, a grey gelding taller than Misty, struck out at me as I pressed the tube into his nose. The tube came out as I ducked back to avoid the sudden explosion of a hoof in my direction.

'He always is a problem. Doug normally uses a twitch. Pablo was the one who bled last time'

Snippets of a Vet's Life

'OK if I use one then?'

'Sure. Whatever it takes. He belongs to Charlotte and she lets him get away with murder. Lucky she is not here because she only gets upset.'

'Who's Charlotte?' I naturally asked.

'My daughter... You'd like her, Rob. I can just tell.'

'I'm sure I would. Now, I'll just get the twitch out of the car,' and gave her daughter no more thought.

The twitch consists of a usually wooden handle, often in the shape of a hammer handle, with at one end, instead of a solid hammerhead, a loop of medium-thickness rope is attached. The operator places a hand through the loop, gently grabbing the horse's upper muzzle and then pulling the hand back, allowing the loop of rope to surround the muzzle. Once in that position, the handle is rotated, which tightens the loop around the muzzle. It sounds barbaric, but it was the accepted method of restraining a non-compliant horse.

I quickly applied the twitch to Pablo, and as expected, he stopped resisting my efforts to drench him. He stood with his head reaching out a bit, and secured by the twitch.

'You could help now if that's possible. Can you hold the twitch?'

While the Matron held the twitch handle, I stood to one side of the horse's head and quickly passed the stomach tube through Pablo's nose and into his gullet or oesophagus. With my free hand, I held up the end with the funnel attached, and the Matron, with her free hand, poured the drench into the funnel. With the flow under gravity, the task of drenching the uncooperative horse was done. Once the tube was out, I released the twitch, and Pablo pulled back slightly in one final display of resistance.

I patted him, and he calmed down. I tied him to the nearest fence.

Success. The job was done, and neither horse had a bloody nose.

'Thanks, Rob. That was great. I think I'll ask for you next time I have any horse work. I'm sure Doug will not mind.'

Having had one of two conversations with Doug over the last few weeks, I inwardly agreed that Doug would not mind.

'Do you remember when I first met you, when you were vaccinating Speedy, my dog, that you said you had a passing interest in opera?'

'Yes. I'm not an opera fan, so I don't know much about it, but I did go once or twice with some friends. And I found it to be enjoyable. Why?'

'Well, I have been so impressed with what you have done today, and what you did for Mr Brown, and I have two spare opera tickets for next week. I can't go, but I wondered if you would like them as a sort of thank-you gift.'

Now that I was no longer a student and could access student pricing, I thought the cost of opera tickets was out of my financial reach, so her offer was an unexpected gift.

But as the old proverb advises, 'Don't look a gift horse in the mouth', I should have perhaps been a bit less forthcoming in my ready acceptance of her offer.

'Yes. That would be wonderful. In fact, fantastic, because I have that weekend off. Thank you, Matron.' I thought this was an unexpected advantage of being a young vet: that people would give me things.

'Good,' she said, paused, and then continued, 'So, um... Would you mind taking my daughter, Charlotte, with you? She also loves the opera. She normally goes with me, and she would be so disappointed to miss out.'

'Ah,' I stumbled before continuing, 'Sure. If she wants to go with me.'

'Oh. She will. Charlotte just loves the Opera,' she gushed, and 'she will like you.'

'OK. I'll be in contact to make the arrangements... with Charlotte. Or...you?'

'Me, Rob. Charlotte is always busy and a bit shy. I want this to be a surprise for her.'

I washed my hands, tipped the water out, and then put the stomach tube, the twitch, and my yellow plastic bucket into the car. I got in, said a quick 'goodbye,' and after negotiating the broken gate and tying it again to the post, left and drove back to the Clinic.

My thoughts lingered on the unmet Charlotte, and I wondered if the Matron had outwitted me or if she was simply generous. So, I was to go on a blind date with Charlotte, whom I had never met. It could be interesting, but I did not mention it to Doug when I returned.

'How was the Matron?' he asked, and, without waiting for a reply, added, 'and how did you go with Pedro?'

'Went well. I had to use a twitch, but I got him done.'

'Well done,' he said, and once again, I rejoiced in his praise.

'And Robbie,' he added, 'Always keep the Matron happy. Always.'

9 – IN THE DEEP END

Friday, at ten-thirty, Jimmy arrived again for coffee and a chat. He always seemed to be at war with somebody, something, or some organisation, and today was no exception.

Doug and I struggled to keep straight faces as he regaled us with his latest run-in with CASA.

'Dougie, Robbie! I can't tell you how stupid they are.'

'Who or what is CASA?' I naturally asked.

'What is CASA? Don't get me started...', at which point Doug interrupted.

'CASA is the Civil Aviation Safety Authority and is the body that regulates Australian aviation safety. And Jimmy hates them with a passion.'

'Safety! Regulates safety! Don't be fooled, Robbie; they know nothing about safety. All they know is how to make bloody regulations. And this latest one is a humdinger!'

He described the new regulation in great detail and with considerable passion, and as I discovered, Jimmy had a disdain for 'regulations' or any constraints in general. He was married to Judy, whom he sometimes called Jude, and from what I could tell, Jimmy spent a lot of his time and energy trying to make sure Judy didn't discover his latest 'project.'

Judy, according to Doug, had also tried to constrain Jimmy over the years.

About a week later, I was having coffee in the Coldstream Supermarket Cafe one Saturday afternoon, quietly reading the paper and luxuriating in being off for the weekend. My reading was suddenly interrupted,

'Hello, Robbie. When you are finished, do you have ten minutes?' I looked up.

'Yes, Jimmy. Why?'

'She's out. I need a hand. Can you help me?'

Jimmy was one of those people who were always ready to assist if anyone else needed a hand. Sometimes, he would help, even when you didn't need a hand. He was that sort of person. He was a community man. He was a 'giver' without any 'strings.' He was constantly enthusiastic and always in a rush about whatever he did. But often he was seemingly angry at somebody or something, but a wicked smile always softened his anger as he related what had recently upset him.

Snippets of a Vet's Life

Except for CASA, which I think he hated with a passion, and he never smiled, even so slightly, when he was discussing them.

It was hard to feel sad or down when you were around Jimmy. He was a good person.

So when Jimmy asked for my help, and notwithstanding that I did not know who 'she' was, I dropped my previous plans for my afternoon off of doing 'nothing' and said,

'Sure. What can I do?'

'We don't have much time, Robbie, so I'll tell you as we drive home. Let's go.'

It transpired that Jimmy had been constructing a fibreglass boat at the back of his house at Sunshine Meadows.

He parked his car on one side of his home and hurried through a break in a large hedge. I followed, quickly walking to keep up. He always had so much energy. At the back of the house was a large lawn that needed mowing and a moderate-sized in-ground swimming pool.

'What do you think, Robbie? She's a beauty, isn't she?'

I was looking at the hull of his new aquatic project. It was fibreglass grey and about 4 metres long by 1.5 metres wide. It rested above the ground on some supports on one side of the pool.

'A boat?...' I said, perplexed, then continued, 'How can I help you?'

'OK, Robbie. We have to test it to see if she's watertight. Before Jude returns, she doesn't understand. Just give me a hand to get it in the pool, will you?'

With some effort, Jimmy and I launched the hull into the water. It sat in the water and appeared not to have any leaks.

'OK, Robbie. Now, jump into it. We have to test it and make sure that it is stable.'

So I jumped in. Jimmy jumped in and, with a push, launched us into the pool's centre. We both stood, I somewhat unsteadily, Jimmy standing as though it was common practice. We stood in the middle of the hull, which proved stable, and it slowly drifted into the centre of the pool.

'OK. Now we have to wait to see if there are any slow leaks...' he said, but before he could continue, an angry woman stormed out the back door and slammed it shut. Was this Judy, I wondered? We both stood bolt upright in the floating boat as though we were two naughty schoolboys caught smoking behind the toilet shed.

'Jimmy! What are you doing?'

The angry woman seemed to ignore me and focused her attention and anger on Jimmy.

Snippets of a Vet's Life

'I told you, Jim, to stop wasting your time on that boat. I go out for 5 minutes, and I come back. What do I find? And who is this?'

She now seemed to realise someone else was standing in the boat.

'Jude. Now Jude. Calm down. Have you met Robbie? He works for Dougie.'

Judy must have realised after spending many years with Jimmy that he always seemed to add to the end of people's names because she then said,

'Hello, Rob.'

I gently leaned down, reached out for the edge, and pulled the boat to the side. Then, carefully stepping out of the boat and onto the pool's edge, I reached out, trying not to slip, and offered my hand to Judy as though greeting her at a garden party.

'A pleasure to meet you, Judy.'

She seemed to discount me as she continued, 'Jimmy. Get that boat out of the pool. There are so many jobs to do around here, and you're playing with boats. Just look at this lawn!'

'Yes, Jude. But we are not playing. More, testing,' he said, looking towards me for affirmation.

And with that, she turned and went inside, again slamming the door. Jimmy furtively smiled at me.

'That was Jude.' There was no further explanation.

A few minutes later, we heard a car drive away. Judy's car, was my guess.

'Quick. Robbie! She's gone! She can get a bit upset. But only if she finds out. Quick, Robbie, jump back into the boat. We have to test for leaks before she comes back. And then we are finished.'

I hesitantly did as he asked. I stood quietly in the centre of the boat, unconsciously looking towards the hills in the distance, and quietly trying to maintain my balance as Jimmy looked for signs of a leak. He was talking about a range of subjects, switching from one to the other as quickly as he took his cigarette out of one side of his mouth and replaced it without interrupting the flow of dialogue.

Then, we heard the not-so-distant sound of a car driving along the driveway.

'Quick, Robbie. She's back. Jude's back! Help me get it out of the pool. There will be hell to pay if she catches us again.' And with that, he jumped to the edge of the pool, which had the unfortunate effect of unbalancing the boat, and I fell into the pool.

He looked at me and said hurriedly, 'Get out! No time for swimming, Robbie,' as I quickly clambered out of the water.

He seemed oblivious of the part he played in my falling into the pool.

Snippets of a Vet's Life

I was now very wet as I helped him get the boat out of the pool. Getting the new craft out was not as easy as getting it in, but we managed to partially place it on the edge. However, we needed to be quicker.

'Jimmy!'

Oops!

'Bugger,' I heard Jimmy say under his breath.

We both looked up like startled kangaroos in a car's headlights.

I was dripping wet with water.

'Why are you still playing with that boat?'

Judy was back and was standing at the back door again. Again, I was ignored by her. She continued, and I could hear in her tone that she was starting to fire up.

'I don't know, Jimmy Dunne. I ask you to do one thing, and... With all this mess around the place...and the lawn still needs to be mowed!'

I thought this was a good time to leave Jimmy, Judy, the boat, and the problem of the unmown lawn, so I excused myself and quietly left. Neither of them seemed to notice.

The following Monday morning, at 10.30 am, Jimmy walked into the clinic for coffee and a chat. He wore on his face his ever-sunny demeanour, and was smoking a cigarette out of the corner of his mouth.

'Your wife seemed a bit, upset?' I said over coffee.

Jimmy's face darkened slightly at the mention of my recent encounter with his wife.

Doug had a slight smile on his face as he said, 'So Robbie, you've met Judy?'

'Yes, over the weekend. I helped launch a small boat in Jimmy's swimming pool. And Judy didn't seem to be very pleased.'

Again, Doug's lack of comment about the boat launching gave the impression that this was not an out-of-the-ordinary activity for Jimmy.

'Nah,' Jimmy said. 'She's happy. That's just Jude. But some things make her unhappy. Has a heart of gold. And Robbie, she loves her horses,' and his face morphed into a wicked smile.

But as Doug later told me, there was a constant 'war' between Judy's love of horses and Jimmy's disdain for them.

And always, the enemy in Jimmy's mind was CASA, and this was not to be the last time I was in a swimming pool, but it was to be the first, that I shared a pool with a donkey.

10 – A NIGHT AT THE OPERA

At the start of the following week, and between clients, I made the call as arranged.

'Now. Matron, is Charlotte still OK going with me to the Opera? I've never actually met Charlotte, and she hasn't met me. It is all a bit…strange?'

'Absolutely, yes! She can't stop talking about it. That's she's going to the opera with you. Can you pick her up from our flat at the back of the hospital, say 6 pm on Friday?'

'Sure. I will have to get off early, but I don't think that will be a problem because Doug is on duty. I'll see you then. Bye.'

I put the phone down and found Doug. He was in the process of desexing a male cat.

'Doug. Can I ask a favour?'

'What is it, Robbie?'

'Would it be possible for me to work longer today or perhaps start earlier tomorrow? I'm willing to work with you, you know.'

'Get to the point, Robbie,' he said tersely, 'and can you put on a pair of sterile gloves and put pressure on the skin bleed?'

It was a command, not a request. I was learning that surgery was not a time for politeness; it was a time for directness, especially if there was a bleed.

'Can I leave earlier than usual to go to the opera on Friday night?'

'The opera? I didn't know you were interested in the opera.'

'Well. The Matron gave me some tickets…'

'Always be careful of the Matron. There are always strings attached,' and while talking, he cut into the testicle, grabbed it and applied constant pressure, stretching the attached chord until it broke and the chord and blood vessel snapped back into the cat's scrotum.

'No. Nothing like that. She very kindly asked me to take her daughter to the opera.' I dabbed a small bleeder automatically.

'So, did she ask you in that way?' He said, but did not look at me as he focused on removing the second testicle.

'Not exactly, but it doesn't matter. I like the opera and can't afford tickets.'

'You do know that Charlotte's boyfriend is the local medico's son, don't you?'

Snippets of a Vet's Life

'No, I didn't.' I quietly reflected to myself, another boyfriend. 'But it's not like we are going on a date or anything like that. She just offered me the tickets, and Charlotte was sort of attached, so I said yes.'

'OK. Yes, you can have the night off. But be careful. The Matron can ruin your reputation if you upset her.'

He released the ties holding the cat's legs in the air and laid the newly desexed cat on its side. We both watched, and then it took a breath.

'Upset who? Charlotte?' I continued.

'No. The Matron!'

He gave the cat an injection of long-acting penicillin and left the room to wash his hands, while Samantha removed the cat from the table and took it to the cat ward to recover.

As arranged, Doug made sure there were no appointments in my name later on Friday afternoon. I drove home to the Green Cottage, had a quick bath in the outside annex to the front verandah that was the bathroom, shaved, put on a bit of underarm deodorant, shined my shoes, and made my way in the car to the Matron's flat at the hospital. I had cleaned the passenger seat and put as much of my vet gear and utensils in the boot as the room allowed. I then wiped the dashboard and generally made my car respectable. I sprayed some car freshener as a final effort to make my car suitable for my passenger and blind date.

I was excited at the thought of meeting Charlotte, whom I had heard by this stage was very attractive, but slightly 'difficult'- whatever that meant.

I knocked. The Matron must have been waiting behind the door because I heard her call out, 'Charlotte? Charlotte? Charlotte, come out, dear. Rob's here.' She said this with a slight nervousness and upward inflection in her voice.

She then opened the door.

'Rob. She's nearly ready. Do you want to come in, and wait inside?'

'If you don't mind, Matron, I'll wait in the car. If we are to arrive at the theatre in plenty of time, we'll need to leave soon. OK?' I was feeling a bit nervous.

I did not go out with many girls when I was at university. Trinity College was an all male residence when I was there, and the only contact I had with girls, out of university lectures, was with the maids who cleaned our rooms, served the meals, and even buttered our toast at breakfast. And, as the College House Keeper, a formidable woman, by the name of Dawn, had warned on entry into college, that the 'maids are OFF LIMITS', whatever that meant.

My home life was a fairly cloistered environment, and friends were not encouraged to visit, mainly because, as my parents explained, they were worried that the horses might injure somebody in our backyard. This sounded believable, but it stifled my learning to be a good host or to be welcoming of friends to my home. Not surprisingly, I became a better guest than host in time.

As I have previously related, I had little contact with girls my age during my teenage years.

I had the regular boyhood infatuations and fantasies, but nothing serious. The closest I came to the opposite sex at school was Saturday night dance classes that the school conducted in the second term of my second-to-last year. At this age, I was a firm believer in the attractive effects that underarm deodorant had, or so I thought, on the opposite sex. So, I always used it a lot, everywhere, before going to dance classes.

And even before picking up Charlotte, I could not pass up a good dose of Old Spice under both arms.

'Here she is,' the Matron announced, looking nervously behind.

A girl about my age pushed past her mother and slammed the door behind her. She was drop-dead beautiful and seemed to know it. Her body and her long blonde hair swayed as she walked towards the car. Her eyes were cold, her mouth set sharp, not broken by any smile. She didn't say a word, but the message was clear: I was an annoyance. And still, I couldn't look away. She had that kind of pull, like standing too close to a lit fuse.

So this was Charlotte, the Matron's daughter.

As she approached the car, I got out and smiled at her.

'Hello,' I said, slightly nervously.

She did not respond. I then went around the other side of the vehicle to open the door for her, but I was too late. My father had taught me the skills of being a 'gentleman'. But to no avail. She got in unassisted and slammed the door shut after her. She looked straight ahead, still with a sour look on her face. I concluded that Charlotte was not happy. In fact, she looked 'pissed off'.

'Hi, Charlotte,' and I nervously added, 'We haven't met. I'm Rob.' I waited for her to respond as I started the car.

But no response was forthcoming from Charlotte.

'OK, then, all settled in, I see. Let's get going. Don't want to be late.'

The Matron had described Charlotte as a bit quiet and somewhat shy. Others, whom I had asked, had said, less generously, she could be 'difficult'.

Perhaps that explained why, for the next 45 minutes of the trip into the city, Charlotte did not utter a word in response to my, at times, effervescent and nervous questions. I did not know what to say in response to her silence, which increasingly worried me.

Snippets of a Vet's Life

Finally, we were waiting at traffic lights and in sight of the Princess Theatre, the venue for that night's opera.

'I want to know only one thing,' Charlotte suddenly said while we waited for the lights to change, staring fiercely ahead..

'Yes?' Perhaps things were improving, I thought.

'How much did my mother pay you to take me out tonight?' she snapped with venom.

Before I could gather my wits and answer her, the lights changed to green and GO, and a car behind me honked its horn impatiently.

'Uh, mm. Nothing. Just the tickets?' I said with a strained voice, unsure of how to respond.

'I thought so,' was all she had to say for the rest of the night.

The following morning, the Matron rang me at home. Early.

'Charlotte had a marvellous time. She couldn't stop talking about you, Rob.'

I now realise that Matron knew how to massage a guy's ego.

'You sure?' I asked, somewhat incredulously. 'That wasn't the impression I got.'

'No? She's a bit shy, and it takes a while to warm up to somebody new.'

'Really?'

'Yes. In fact, Charlotte asked if you could come to dinner...perhaps a Sunday night in two or three weeks? I told her I would ask. Is that a yes?'

'You sure? About Charlotte. I mean...She seemed a bit angry with me...'

'Just shy, Rob. You know how girls can be. See you at 6 pm. Bye'

With that, I was destined for another meeting with Charlotte, and this time with her mother. And I reflected that I did not know much about girls, as the Matron had wrongly assumed.

And I knew even less about their mothers.

11 – ONE PLUS TWO DEATHS

'You'll be right, Robbie,' Jimmy added as he washed his cup in preparation for leaving. 'Don't doubt yourself. Just do it as though Doug was watching and helping,' he said to help me.

'Thanks, Jimmy. Yep, you are right. I can do this. I have given a lot of cats intravenous injections, so it should be easy.'

'That's it, Robbie. You will manage. See you,' and he left.

But even though I professed confidence, I was not confident. Hitting the cephalic or arm vein in a cat, especially if they are not cooperative, can be very difficult, and usually, you only have one go. I was not consoled by the obvious: that most cats have two arms, so if I failed with the first attempt, I could always move to the other arm. However, having once failed, there was a good chance that the second attempt would fail.

I felt nervous.

When I was young, as a boy, I was relatively carefree. I did not have many stressors in my life except the normal ones: my two older brothers, both of whom called me 'Rat' as a nickname and my parents, who, as I was to learn later, had their own relationship problems. But not much bothered me. And, even as I progressed through school, I maintained a lightheartedness, and not much truly troubled me. Until one day in church, when I was about 14 years old, being confirmed into the brotherhood of the Church, and sitting at the front of what I remember to be a large congregation, but in reality was not, I suddenly needed to go to the toilet, to urinate. I was busting. I had gone before the service started, so I was surprised by the situation.

But leaving would have been embarrassing, so I held on as best as I could. There is nothing more focusing than a bladder that is getting fuller. I did not listen at all to what was said. My thoughts were on my bladder, and if God was all-forgiving and comforting, why did I want to go to the toilet? Why just now? Where was God when I truly needed him? Where was his mercy? Finally, I just had to go. So, I stood up and quickly walked from the front pew to the back door along the central aisle, feeling as if all eyes were on me. Puberty probably didn't help. Most kids go through an embarrassing phase, so in that regard, I was normal. But what many would just brush off, I couldn't. I over-analysed. The pending end-of-year exams probably did not help. I was stressed.

And as I learnt when I went to the doctor the following day, I had a urinary tract infection, hence the feeling of urgency.

Snippets of a Vet's Life

And then something truly weird happened. It occurred to my very logical brain that there were other situations where a person, that is, me, just can't always attend to an urgent call of nature. For example, sitting in a car at traffic lights, waiting for green, and sitting in an aeroplane waiting for the take-off to start, with the restriction that 'all seat belts must remain buckled until the light goes off', or marching in line at school, or... I started to sweat as I realised there were many situations where I was not in control, and I couldn't go to the toilet if needed. The following week, I had what was to be the first of many panic attacks, and I thought I was going to die. But I did not. And so began the unconscious creation of a new me, someone who needed to be in control so that I could feel I could leave if necessary. I projected confidence, but I was always hiding insecurity. For some people, because of my need to control, I probably became a pain in the proverbial backside.

My thoughts returned to what I needed to do today: to hit the vein as Samantha showed the old couple with their cat into the examination room. Puddles was wrapped in the old lady's arms.

'Come in,' I said in my most confident voice. This won't take long. I'm Dr Rob. Doug has explained the situation: We need to end Puddle's life, and he apologises for not being here to send Puddle on her way.'

And then I stopped, reflecting that perhaps I was talking too much. I was stressed and worried about being unable to hit the arm vein.

The older man had his arm around her shoulder. He held her gently. They stood together, both slightly bent over, perhaps a bit crushed by the situation. I could see they were a team. He comforted her. She looked down at Puddles, encased in a towel held gently in her arms.

'Hello, Dr. Rob,' he said, looking at me. As he said it, I felt a slight discomfort in being addressed as 'doctor' by this old man. Their quiet presence radiated a calmness, even though it was not a calm situation.

'Thank you for stepping in. Doug has been wonderful with Puddles, and we knew when we got the phone call on Friday that Puddles' time was up. He hasn't eaten for days, and I am thankful that Doug called us. And now Dr Rob, we are in your hands.'

By now, I was feeling very uncomfortable with the doctor's title, so I said, 'Just call me Rob.' And then, like many young vets, when faced with a stressful situation, I retreated into the facade of being the vet: in control, knowledgeable, and needing to express my knowledge, devoid of emotion.

'I have looked at the report and the blood results, and there is nothing else we can do. When the kidneys are gone, animals feel sick. And that explains why she has been vomiting over the last few weeks, and apart from using intravenous fluids to wash the waste products out of her system...' and before I could continue in this monologue displaying how much I knew, he interrupted me with, 'That's OK, Rob. We know about kidney disease. Our only son died from it last year. We have struggled for years with Richard's situation. He was so sick, and we saw how it affected him, so there is no need for you to explain kidney disease. We had to watch him decline and eventually die. It was terrible.'

My face flushed. I felt embarrassed at my brashness, my need to be the vet, and the one in control. For once, I stopped and thought, contemplated their grief, and felt I had no proper understanding or training to handle this situation. It was the start of me realising that to be a good vet, I needed to know more about an owner than their name.

I simply said, 'I'm sorry. I didn't know,' and added, 'I simply don't know what to say except sorry.'

'That's OK. We don't make a lot of it. We just get on. But...before you...,' and he reached out to hold his wife's hand, 'Can we have some time by ourselves with Puddles?'

'Yes, certainly. I'll just be outside. Have as long as you need.' I said, and I left the room.

I stood outside the closed door. I heard her cry. I had no training in handling these situations. I knew death as an intellectual concept, but I had little contact with dying, except for my grandmother, who died when I was a vet student.

My thoughts were interrupted by the sound of the examination room door opening.

'We are ready.'

'Samantha, can you give me a hand?'

In caring for people and their emotions, Samantha was much more experienced.

'How long have you had her?' she asked gently.

'A long time. She was really our son's cat, and when he came to live with us again a few years ago, she came with him.'

'She was your son's cat?'

'Yes,' said the old woman, lifting her head and looking at us for the first time. 'Puddles was his. We are doing this for Richard.'

Again, I didn't know what to say, but Samantha did. As I listened, I realised that Samantha was wiser than her years. Perhaps she had been through it with Doug many times.

'Then let's end her suffering. Deciding to end her life is, in a way, your last gift to Puddles for all the years of joy that she gave your son and you.'

They both looked at Samantha and then at me.

'When you are ready,' Samantha gently directed, 'just hand her to me, and Rob and I will care for her.'

Snippets of a Vet's Life

There was a pause. They looked at each other, and then the older lady handed her precious bundle into the care of Samantha's outstretched hands.

'It's time,' he said, 'Go ahead.'

Samantha placed Puddles gently on the examination table. I could see that what she had was that she 'cared.' I, however, retreated into being the professional and directed her to hold Puddles' leg out in front. I held the paw for support, clipped the hair over the vein, and dabbed some alcohol onto the skin, not to sterilise it, but to assist me in seeing the vein underneath the thin skin of Puddles' right arm.

Without being told, Samantha gently put her elongated thumb over the vein at the top of the leg. The back pressure caused the vein to become inflated with blood that could not escape.

Perhaps because I was concerned for them, and not fixated on failing at what I had to achieve, I felt calm, and without any feelings of anxiety, I gently pushed a small needle into the vein and, looking at them, asked, 'Are you ready?'

The old man said quietly, 'Yes,' and the old lady quietly started to weep.

And with that permission, I gently pushed the plunger into the body of the syringe. The green drug entered her vein and, a second later, the overdose of phenobarbitone, an anaesthetic, for that was what was in the syringe, calmly ended Puddle's life.

She lay limp on the towel. Lifeless. She was gone.

Sometimes, after death from intravenous injection, an animal can take a big final breath. It is the ancient reptilian part of the brain attempting to kick-start 'life', and I had been taught that it could alarm owners if it happened.

I removed the syringe and quietly told them that even though she had 'gone', she may take a final deep breath. I reassured them that this final breath was not an indication of coming back to life but the final sign of death.

There was quiet in the room, and I said, 'Stay in here for as long as you need. And when you are finished, leave her, and we will take care of her.'

'Thanks, Rob. But we want to take her with us. When Richard died, we planted a tree, and we are going to bury her next to that tree.'

I realised that I should have asked this question much earlier instead of making an assumption, but no harm; I did learn.

As if a load had been lifted from his shoulders, he stood more erect and had a presence about him that I had not earlier seen. He turned to Samantha, standing quietly in the corner and asked for Puddles to be wrapped in a blanket.

Snippets of a Vet's Life

'Is there anything we can do for you?' I asked I was still emotionally out of my depth, but I thought it was the right thing to offer.

'That's very kind of you, but we have been preparing for this day. We will be OK. Thank you.'

I watched them leave with their precious bundle and wondered about their grief.

And a few days later, I received my first thank-you card.

'Dear Dr Rob,

Thank you for all the care you extended to my wife and me. We cannot thank you enough. And please let Samantha know that her words that it was our last gift to Puddles were incredibly heartfelt because we did feel guilty at ending her life early.

We are now both at peace after burying Puddles at the base of Richard's tree.

With much thanks.

And perhaps, one day, we might cross paths again.

Regards,

Robert and Mary Jones.'

Two weeks later, they died after their car crashed, for no apparent reason, late one afternoon, into a tree on a quiet back road.

Rod Graham

12 – HILLARY AND HANNAH THE HEN

'Good morning,' I said, addressing the young girl. 'And who have we here?' I asked, looking at the hen she was holding in a towel.

'Hannah, with two H's and two N's,' came the rapid response, and I had to pause as I mentally considered what she had said.

'Hannah, I got it. I'm Rob, with one r,' I said, picking up on her name comment, and then asked, 'And what's your name?'

'Hillary? With two L's. Are you a real doctor?' she responded rapidly.

'No, and yes. I'm not a person doctor, but I'm an animal doctor. '

'Now, Hillary, not too many questions,' her mother said. 'She is very advanced for her age and can ask and ask. She loves spelling.'

'Thanks. But I'm OK with questions. And I have one for you: What brings you here today?'

Snippets of a Vet's Life

'We are worried about Hannah. She's gone limp. She was OK yesterday, but this morning....'

Hillary carefully unbounded Hannah, the hen, from a towel and placed her on the examination table.

The hen sat where she had been placed. Her head slowly dropped until it was resting on the tabletop. Her eyelids drooped, and she hunched her back as though attempting to hold up her wings.

'Do you have any other chooks or just Hannah?' I asked the mother.

'No. Just Hannah.'

This response was quickly followed by Hillary asking, 'Is she dying?'

I was slightly stunned by the directness of her question.

'Well... I have to see what's wrong first. I need to examine her and ask some more questions,' I said to deflect her confronting question and give me time to think.

As students, we had a few lectures on poultry diseases. Hannah was the first hen I had seen as a qualified vet, so I was scrambling as I looked at Hannah, the hen. She just sat on the table, wings dropped, hunched back, and comb flaccid.

'How was she last week?'

'Seemed to be OK. She has her cage outside. It's a big cage, and she lives in it. We live on a farm, and there are foxes.'

'Do foxes eat chooks?' Hillary said, interrupting her mother.

I was about to respond with a positive. But, I hesitated as I did not wish to alarm the child.

'Why do you ask?' By asking a question, I felt somewhat more in control of the conversation.

I was pleased that I had learnt to use a deflecting question. Doug, my boos was the source of this knowledge. His advice had been to ask back a question if I was presented with something I could not or should not answer.

'My brother told me.'

'Oh,' was all I could respond. I was a bit stumped for a response. I realised I had to practice this new skill of asking deflecting questions. I retreated once again to the safety of a young vet by asking questions about a case's history.

'So, she has been OK. Is she eating?'

'Yes. Hillary feeds her every day,' said the mother.

'And do you feed her chook food?'

'Yes. Is that a problem?'

'No. Not normally. When did you buy the bag? A new bag?'

Snippets of a Vet's Life

'About two weeks ago. It seems to be OK. It's what we've always fed her.'

'And yesterday, she was alright?' I was running out of things to ask, so I reverted to another of a young vet's safety behaviours and started to examine the flaccid fowl.

'Her eyelids are drooping. Just today?'

While the mother and I talked, Hillary was exploring the room. Out of the corner of my eye, I saw she was about to open the drug cupboard.

'Oops. No, you mustn't do that,' I said.

'Hillary, come back. Close that door, and behave,' said the mother. The girl obediently did as she was told, returned to the table, and started to caress the limp hen's head.

'Is she drinking?' I asked, returning to my questioning and feeling lost for possible diagnoses.

'I think so. I fill her water bowl every morning and haven't noticed any change.'

'And today?'

'I didn't notice. I found her huddled in the corner.

'I saw a fox near her,' the girl said.

'You saw a fox?' I asked.

'Hillary! Stop making up stories! ' The mother said, and then, directing her attention to me, explained, 'She can be very creative sometimes. I'm sorry.'

'No problem. When did you see a fox, Hillary?'

'Last night. I heard it. So, I went outside.'

'And was there a fox?'

'Yes, but I saw it run away. Hannah was in the corner, so I gave her some food.'

'You fed her?' her mother asked, somewhat surprised.

'Yes. The possums didn't want the food, so I gave it to Hannah. She gobbled it up.'

The mother sheepishly explained, 'To stop possums from eating our roses, I have been putting food scraps on a plate, but not for a few days. I noticed that they had stopped eating the food recently.'

'And you fed those scraps to Hannah, Hillary?'

'Yes. And the maggots.'

'Maggots, with two G's?' I asked, once again returning to our game to engage her.

She smiled at our game and added, 'The fox ran away. The possums, with three S's, didn't want it, so I gave it to Hannah.'

'And she gobbled it up, and that's with two B's?' I asked.

'Yes. All of it.'

'And are there maggots in it?'

'Yes. She ate the maggots first and then the scraps.'

Now addressing the mother, I asked, 'About how long ago did you put the food out for the possums?'

'A few days. After dinner one night. I just put the scraps out straight off the plates.'

'With the warm weather, I'm not surprised that there were a few maggots.'

'Are maggots bad for Hannah?' asked Hillary.

'No. Hens can eat many different living things, including slugs, snails, and small lizards.'

'Yuck. I ate a slug. Ugh, I spat it out.'

Her statement reminded me how, as a child, I had once picked a cigarette butt off the road and eaten it. I felt sick for a few hours. But I never ate a slug. I returned my gaze to the sick hen. Mentally, I ticked a few boxes- dropped wings, her comb not erect, eyelids closed, head down, sudden onset after eating food that may have been off and rotting, and maggot ingestion.

All this in the time it took Hillary to come up with her next, confronting question.

'Will she die?' she asked, her voice filled with pleading.

And I was able to answer truthfully, 'Probably not. I think I know what's wrong with her. Botulism!' I pronounced it with an inner sense of outstanding achievement. 'I am sure. Botulism spores are everywhere. In the soil, on dead leaves, and even in the poo of wild birds,'

'Poo! Poo! Mummy, he said, poo!'

'Hillary. Let him speak. He's a vet. He can say poo.'

'Not fair!' she snapped back, in a sulk.

'Sorry about 'poo' The proper word is faeces,' and I spelled it out for her. 'But I like saying the naughty 'P' word whenever I can,' and I smiled at her to re-engage. It worked. She smiled back.

'Can you tell me more about botulism?' the mother asked, returning us to the hen.

'For the spores to reproduce, they require a warm, moist and low oxygen environment like upturned compost or rotting food scraps. And as grow, they release a deadly neurotoxin. Hannah has eaten some of this toxin in the old food, and the toxin has travelled to her nerves, causing the paralysis. Maggots can also eat the spores; the toxin is produced inside them, and Hannah ate the maggots. Therefore, I am fairly certain that she has botulism.'

'Can it be treated...or...,' the mother asked, leaving the obvious unsaid.

'I think so. I will have to look this disease up in one of my books. It's the first time I have seen it,' or for that matter, the first time I had treated a hen, but I thought it best not to reveal that bit of information.

I left the room and noticed two people were waiting for me in the waiting room. I glanced at Samantha with an unsaid, 'Why didn't you let me know that they were waiting?' look. But she ignored me.

Something was up with her, I thought. Clients who have to wait, can become angry.

I quickly scanned my poultry lecture notes and was pleased to find a mention of botulism in poultry and its treatment. However, I also noted that the prognosis, or expected outcome, was poor. Reading the notes, I saw botulism in a new light. It is not an infection of the body with the bacteria Clostridium botulinum that causes the disease; rather, it is the ingestion of the neurotoxin that the bacteria produce when rotting food or decaying vegetation is consumed that causes the disease.

Fully armed with knowledge, I returned to the examination room and, on the way, indicated to the waiting clients that I would only be a bit longer.

'OK. What we have to do is admit her for a few days, and the first thing I will do is give her a dose of charcoal powder to soak up any toxins that may still be in her digestive system and then flush her insides using molasses in water.'

'Is there an antidote?' asked the mother.

'No. There is nothing specific, just supportive care until Hannah can detoxify the neurotoxin. Let's see how she is tomorrow, and I'll call you.'

'On Sunday?' the mother asked, surprised.

'I'm on duty, so I'll be taking care of her. Any other questions?'

'Will she die?' asked Hillary, once again.

'If we can get her through the next 48 hours, there is a good chance she will live. If there are no further questions, I will take her out the back, and the nurse will make her as comfortable as possible.

I'm happy to report that Hannah recovered to cluck another day.

And the waiting clients were not angry.

13 – MRS PRIDHAM'S CLOCK

For some weeks, I slept on a mattress on the floor of the Green Cottage kitchen. It was not ideal, but it was much better than spending my nights on a camp stretcher and sharing a room with sick or distressed dogs at the clinic.

The door into the sitting room was wedged shut by the wooden supports having collapsed over the years. Not long after taking over the Green Cottage, I crawled beneath it and inspected the supports. The problem quickly became apparent. The central fireplace and chimney structure rested on firm concrete foundations. But many of the wooden stumps that supported the walls and floor had rotted, and many had partially collapsed into the underlying soil, causing parts of the cottage and the floor to drop around the central fireplace, like a partially collapsing umbrella.

This was why the door between the kitchen and the living room would not open. Using a car jack, I planned to lift the sunken parts around the fireplace, which would give access to the living room. My plan then was to gradually lift the cottage with a car jack and replace the rotted stumps with bricks.

And this is what I had been doing on this particular Saturday, my day off from work. That evening, for the first time, after a lot of car jacking under the floorboards, I could open the stuck door and enter the sitting room. The sitting room formed the centre part of the cottage, and a fireplace on the other side of the kitchen stove dominated it. The room had two comfortable sitting chairs, and along the wall opposite the fireplace was a cloth couch. The floor was covered in part by a green rug. And there was dust.

Through a large window, I could see the adjacent paddock, and on the other side of the sitting room was a doorway that led into a dining room. The room was dominated by a large wooden dining table, the top of which was covered in dust. I wiped part of the tabletop with a cloth, revealing a polished surface. Around the table were eight dining room wooden chairs with cloth seats and backs, also covered in dust. It was as though I was looking back in time. And considering how hard it had been for me to enter this part of the cottage, I wondered how long ago this room had witnessed a dinner. The table was old and grand; I suspected it had come from the main house at some stage.

On the other side of the sitting room, opposite the kitchen door, was a door that led into a short passageway to the still-stuck front door. With an effort,

Snippets of a Vet's Life

I was able to open the passage door, but not the front door. I realised at some stage that I would need to jack up the foundations under this area. Once through and into the passage, there were two bedrooms, one on either side of the central passage. I moved my mattress into one of the front bedrooms.

I have always struggled to get to sleep, and on this particular night, the first night that I slept in my new bedroom, I once again struggled. I was excited about the whole scenario: I had fallen into a great job with a good boss, a beautiful country area not too far from Melbourne, a cottage to live in, and five acres for a horse. And, all this for a peppercorn rent a year. I had been lucky.

Now, when I have trouble sleeping, I simply get out of bed, read a book for 15 minutes, and then return to bed, which often resolves the problem.

However, I had not yet learned this trick at this stage in my life, and on that particular night, I found myself still wide awake and restless at about 2:00 am.

I heard a bell chime. I knew that it was coming from the direction of Emmerton House. I waited for a second chime. There was no second chime. I waited.

And I waited. There were no more chimes.

I lay restless for the next hour, and the clock again chimed. And once again, I counted. First one, then another, and then a third. I eventually went to sleep.

Rod Graham

The next night, I was again visited by restlessness, and again, at 2:00 a.m., I heard a chime. I waited again, but there was no second chime. I waited longer, but there were no more chimes. I lay there for a while, still wide awake, and wondered about the chimes. Why was there no second chime for 2:00 am?

By this stage, I recalled that there was a bell tower above the old stable block to the side of Emmerton House. The hourly tolling of the bell was coming from this bell tower. I waited until 3:00 am and heard three bell chimes. There was a problem clearly with 2:00 am.

Part of my agreement with Mrs Pridham, my landlady, was never to telephone her, but there was no prohibition on writing her a letter. That is what she had requested when I was given the use of the Cottage. I rolled out of bed, sat at my desk, and, over the next two hours, wrote the following letter,

Dear Mrs Pridham,

As Winter beckons Spring, itself an invitation to Summer, my thoughts briefly dwell upon this changing masterpiece. And I have concluded that she, the one we call Nature, relies most heavily upon those changing chimes that Emmerton hourly chants.

But alas!

This year, Winter will not know when to end or Spring to descend since those chimes from that clock aren't quite what they ought to be.

Snippets of a Vet's Life

Rob McBride.

And, later that day, I gave it to the postmistress of the local post office to put in the Emmerton House post box.

Two days later, I went into the Coldstream Post Office to pick up my letters, and the post lady commented as I was about to leave: 'That must have been an interesting letter you wrote to Mrs Pridham. She was in here this morning and, after reading your letter, exclaimed to nobody in particular, 'Oh, dear. The poor boy has lost his mind in that Cottage!'

The post lady then reported that Mrs Pridham reread my letter and excused herself, saying, 'I have to go.'

About a week after my letter, I received a letter that was hand-delivered to the vet clinic before I arrived for work.

Dear Dr McBride,

Hark. Listen and hear!

Two and two again do meet in the Night and the Morn.

Pamela Pridham.

And so started a correspondence that ebbed and flowed over the next ten years.

Most, but not all, of her letters to me have sadly been lost. And perhaps my letters to her were probably quickly dispatched to the waste bin.

Rod Graham

That night, I fell asleep while waiting to hear the chimes for 2:00 am.

14 – A CLIENT COMPLAINS

On my way to work, I stopped at the local service station for coffee and toast, and so I arrived well-nourished and in time for the start of the workday. Rain had fallen overnight, the air was crisp, and the new day seemed promising.

I felt at peace with the world, but the feeling was not to last.

I parked, enthusiastically bounded up the clinic steps, and entered our waiting room. I was early. The doorbell had just stopped ringing when I was greeted with a short command.

'Doug wants to see you,' Samantha said before I could say good morning. She still seemed a bit negative toward me. I was starting to realise that she didn't like me, and if I was honest, I did not particularly like her. We tolerated each other.

'He's in?' I said, trying to put warmth in my voice. Doug rarely arrived before 9:00 am.

'Yep. Early call.'

Doug had been on duty the night before, and I had used my free time to go to the local picture theatre.

'Rob!' he said in greeting, with a slightly dark look. What had happened to the usual, Robbie, I wondered.

'Good morning, Doug. Samantha said that you wanted to see me.'

'Mrs Spearmint called me at home early this morning and was very upset. Did you tell her last night that the dog would be OK despite vomiting all day yesterday?'

'Well, no...and yes. She rang just as we closed last night. She wanted to come in because she was worried about her dog. I asked her how long it would take to get to the clinic, and she replied that it would be about 30 minutes. I explained that we were closing and that because I was going out, I couldn't wait.'

'So, you told her that you couldn't wait?'

'Well, yes, but I questioned her about her dog, which sounded like a simple gastro. She told me they lived on a farm. While talking, I looked up her record card and saw that her dog had a history of eating garbage. You've treated it a few times. Sounded like another episode of the same. I told her I thought it could wait until the morning.'

'So, Rob, let me get this clear. You told her to wait until the morning and not to worry?'

'Sort of.' I was starting to get uncomfortable with his continuing interrogation.

Snippets of a Vet's Life

'A vomiting dog? Wait until the morning? And DON'T WORRY! Robbie, that was the wrong call.'

I could tell he was trying to control his anger. This was a side of my employer I had never experienced before.

'Why do you think she called us?' he asked.

'Because the dog had been vomiting… all day,' I said in my defence, subtly suggesting that the client was at fault for waiting so long to call us.

'Well, she was worried! And that's why she called us. She was WORRIED!'

'But I told her to call back if there was a problem, and that you were on duty.'

'She didn't want to bother us. That was the effect of what you said. She stayed up all night with the dog. She called me early this morning. I told her to come straight in. The dog was very flat when I eventually saw it. Sick. Probably dehydrated because of the vomiting'

'It's here?' and then added, attempting to lessen my guilt, 'I'm sorry. I didn't know. I thought it would wait.'

'Wait! Robbie, I've admitted her dog, and you and I will be operating on it this morning. I am suspicious that it has a foreign body lodged in its abdomen. She is angry with you, and I have to admit, I am as well.'

'Why angry? Sorry, but Doug, I told her to contact us if it gets worse. What else should I have done?' in a failing attempt to defend myself.

'You should have seen the dog last night!'

'But I was going out. I had booked a ticket to the movies,' and as I said the words, I realised it was the wrong thing to say.

He went silent and had a very dark look on his face. I waited, unsure of what to say next and how to placate him.

'Robbie, you have a lot to learn,' he said, taking a few deep breaths before continuing. 'A client always comes first,' he added, 'even if you are …going to the movies.' He said the last words with an edge, and I could tell he was very angry with me. It was the first time that I had upset him.

He turned and was about to leave when he added a final insult, 'She thought that you didn't care. And that Robbie, if she is right, really angers and disappoints me!'

Now I felt angry. I did care. I wasn't going to be on duty; Doug was. I had done the right thing by telling the client to call if there were any problems later.

And I formed an internal narrative that she had probably distorted what I said. My boss had not defended me. He seemed to believe her, not me. I felt unsupported.

I felt that I was almost the victim! I thought he was unfair, unjust, and unkind, along with all the other emotions that a new clinician feels when caught out wrong. For the first time, I disliked a client and saw my boss in a slightly different light. I felt unsupported.

I still had much to learn about myself and my emotions; others sometimes saw the world and me differently from what I thought.

The university had trained me in veterinary knowledge, but some wisdom was to come much later.

The surgery was scheduled at 10:30 am. Samantha rang and told Jimmy not to come that morning. Besides the routine desexing of dogs, cats, and a randy rabbit, I had not assisted Doug with any more complex surgery. I judged him to be a confident surgeon who performed what was necessary efficiently.

But Juno's surgery was a bigger task.

Juno was the name of the Labrador who had been vomiting intermittently over the last 24 hours. We both lifted the sedated dog onto the surgery table.

He rested quietly on his sternum and chest. I stood on his side, reached over his top, and put my thumb across the centre of his right front leg. At the same time, I lay gently on his back to restrain him as Doug injected the anaesthetic drug into the cephalic vein in his arm. There was no struggle, and he quietly slumped into an induced sleep. He stopped breathing. I was slightly worried.

But this was normal at the start of a general anaesthetic in the days when we used Thiopentone to induce and maintain an anaesthetic. I knew the science, but I felt uneasy.

Doug was calm.

Then Juno took a breath, and then, seconds later, another. From then on, he quietly breathed.

Samantha, who had been standing to one side while Juno was induced, then stepped forward. Together, we rolled the recumbent Juno on his back. We put sandbags on either side of his chest to keep him with his abdomen uppermost, and his legs in the air.

'Robbie. You OK with keeping an eye on him while I prep up?'

Doug left the room, and minutes later returned in a green surgical gown and sterile latex gloves. Juno quietly kept breathing as Samantha shaved his abdomen and then sterilised the skin using a mixture of methylated spirits and chlorhexidine. The nurse made a final few longitudinal swipes along the abdominal skin using sterile swabs soaked in iodine. She then adjusted the surgical light to shine on the intended incision site. All this happened without Doug issuing any directions or Samantha asking any questions. They were obviously a team, and I reflected that perhaps some of Samantha's antagonism to me may have been that I was intruding into her domain.

Juno was ready. Doug waited patiently while Samantha went about her tasks.

Snippets of a Vet's Life

Then, with a simple 'Ready,' he stood at the edge of the table, and Samantha, holding the outside of a sterile pack, handed him a green sterile drape that he took from the inside, maintaining sterility.

He then draped one side of the abdomen and, with the next green cotton sheet, draped the other side. He stabilised the drapes by attaching them to the skin using sharp clamps that grabbed the skin through the drape material.

Again, they worked as a team while I monitored the anaesthetic. I counted Juno's breaths; they were even. Without asking, I realised that Samantha had previously monitored the anaesthetic. I could see why she may have sensed me as an unwelcome intruder.

This was an era when vets trained their own surgical staff on-site. No post-school colleges were yet training veterinary nurses ready for the veterinary workplace.

And close bonds naturally developed between the nurse and the vet, who often had been their teacher.

With a steady and experienced hand, Doug made an incision along the centre of the abdomen and then a second incision through the underlying muscle layers until he was over the peritoneum. This thin fibrous layer guarded the entrance to the intestines. With a pair of sharp surgical scissors in one hand and tissue forceps in the other, he pulled the peritoneum up, made a slight nip through it, and then, having gained an entrance, used the scissors to widen the incision. By doing so, he exposed the abdominal contents.

The whole process of safely opening the abdominal cavity was performed quickly and in silence.

'Samantha. Can you get that bleeder?'

Using a sterile swab and not directly touching the wound with her fingers, she applied pressure to part of the incised skin that was oozing a bit of blood. After about thirty seconds, she removed her hand and looked; it was still oozing. She reapplied pressure, waited, and removed the swab; the oozing had stopped this time.

Doug used his gloved hands to feel inside Juno's abdomen, gently palpating the intestines. And, as if his hands were in a can of large worms, the intestine would fall back into place once he moved from one section to the next.

'OK. Robbie, have a look here,' and I directed my sight to where he indicated.

He showed me a section of intestine that was slightly engorged with blood and larger than the intestines on either side.

'Is the lump solid?' I asked.

'Yes. It feels like…perhaps…' and as he talked, he felt around the lump, 'part of a corn kernel. I will need you to glove up and assist me, and Samantha, you do your normal job monitoring the anaesthetic.'

Snippets of a Vet's Life

So, I was correct. I had supplanted one of Samantha's roles. I wondered what other tasks I had taken over that had been part of her job.

I washed my hands in the special surgical soap and dried them using a sterilised towel. Then, I rewashed them in chlorhexidine hand wash and dried them using a new sterilised towel. Samantha then handed me the first open sterile glove inside a sterile pack, then the other, and now, using the already gloved hand, I finished pulling the second glove onto my other hand.

I was ready.

I stood across the table from Doug. To maintain sterility, I held my gloved hands together as if in prayer. I learned this posture at veterinary school, and it was an accepted way to ensure that the sterile gloves or hands would not unconsciously touch unsterile surfaces.

'OK. Good. Now, Robbie, I want you to pull the edges of the incision apart using the retractors to give me better access to the abdomen.' I had done this before as a vet student.

'That's good. Just hold them in that position.'

I did as he directed. He quickly pulled the intestine through the incision, placing the exteriorised intestine on the sterile drape surrounding the incision site.

'Ok. You can release the retractors.'

I did as he directed, and the incision gently closed around the base of the exposed intestine.

He then made a small stab incision into the wall of the intestine, and at the start of where the intestines were slightly swollen. A small quantity of intestinal fluid escaped from the hole he had just made, and he put a plastic kidney-shaped dish under the area to catch any more fluid that flowed.

'OK, Robbie. Can you swab the area?'

I did as he asked and then discarded the used gauze.

Using the same scissors with which he had created the stab incisor, Doug extended the incision along the length of the swollen intestine, making his cut just long enough for him to grab the end of the protruding corn cob with forceps. With gentle pressure, he could remove the cob from the intestines and onto the edge of the surgery table.

'That came out easily, Robbie. What do you think?'

'Great. Are you now going to close?'

'No. You are. First, I will flush the area with saline solution to remove any intestinal contents that may have leaked out. So, I need you to let go of the retractors, just lay them down, and then Samantha will hand you a pack with sterile gauze inside it. Take the gauze from inside the pack and dab each around the intestine incision, and then, after each dab, discard the swab. That way, you won't spread bacteria from inside the intestines into the surrounding area.'

Snippets of a Vet's Life

'OK. I understand,' I said, thinking he told me what was evident to a trained vet.

I did as he asked, and, as I was so engaged, he discarded the gloves he had worn for a new sterile pair.

Using his hands, gloved again in sterile gloves, he used his fingers to hold the incision site apart.

'Now, Robbie. Have you ever closed an intestinal incision before?'

'No. But I have watched it being done many times in training. I've learnt the principles.'

'OK. I'll watch as you stitch.'

Using sterile forceps, I first picked up one edge of the cut intestine and gently pushed a surgical needle through it, with the suture material attached. Then, I picked up the opposing edge and threaded the needle through that. Holding the end of the suture material in one hand, with the other end held by the needle pusher, I created a loose knot to ensure the opposing edges of the intestine were aligned.

'That's good, Robbie. Now, not too tight.'

Then, I repeated the move and created a second knot. This time, the knot was tighter, closing down on the first knot and ensuring it would not 'slip'.

'Good Robbie. Now do one final knot just to be sure.' And I did.

I knew what to do. I had assisted surgeons many times during my training at the vet school, but Doug's positive encouragement made me feel proud of my achievement.

Doug swabbed the area with wet swabs, keeping the area free of oozing blood. And I continued until the intestines were intact again.

'Don't close the skin yet. Before you do, I want to check that the closure is tight and not leaking.'

And with that, he gently gathered in one hand part of the intestine that was closer to the stomach and, with a milking action, forced the contents into the area that I had surgically closed.

And we both saw a small leak where I had placed the first stitch.

'OK, Robbie. Remove that stitch and redo it. And Samantha, before he does that, use a sterile swab to clean the area.'

We followed his directions, and this time, there was no leakage.

'Always test your work, Robbie. What may appear to be a tight closure sometimes isn't. Overall, you have done well for your first intestinal closing.'

I closed the skin with simple, interrupted sutures as though I were repairing a rip in a cotton sheet.

'Now remember one thing, Robbie. The owner will always judge your work, initially not by the outcome but by how neat the skin stitches are. So always make them neat and equal, but do not forget that somebody has to remove them. So always leave the ends long enough to snip under the knot to remove the stitch easily. OK?'

Doug moved our patient off the table and placed him in the recovery cage, with the door open.

Although Juno weighed over 30 kg, Doug lifted him effortlessly. Later, I learned that he had been a school rugby player.

'Doug. I know that the area was not sterile because of some leakage of intestinal contents. Should we be worried about that?'

'What you have learnt is probably correct, but what I am teaching you is practical. And as you will learn, the practice of veterinary science, in the real world, is an ongoing negotiation with...' and a slight smile softened his face as he quietly said, 'with God. One day, you will understand. Robbie. It is us... against God.'

And then he added, with a wry smile, 'And, of course, a good shot of penicillin and a follow-up course of antibiotic tablets will also help!'

15 – WE ARE HERE TO HELP YOU, MADAM

He leaned back in the chair and continued with his hands behind his head.

'So, overall, Robbie, you are doing a good job. You seem to have a natural flair for the horse clients, and they like you. I'm glad because horse work doesn't enthuse me. I just don't like horses.'

He paused, and then with a slight smile, added, 'And as you know, they can sometimes, kick!'

He was referring to the time a few weeks earlier when he had asked me to attend to his mother's horse, and it had kicked me in the groin, causing me to pass out. I looked back at him with a feigned look of hurt, remembering the three days off he had given me to recover, and then smiled at his comment.

'Yes. Some of them can ... kick,' I said, sagely nodding.

We had met for breakfast in the local roadhouse. I was interested in how my boss thought I was doing in my first year. He had become angry with me a few times recently. And he was usually a calm person.

He continued, 'My only concern is that sometimes you appear to put your needs before the clients and their problems. And that's a poor attitude.'

I bristled a bit, but contained my thoughts. After all, I had asked for his feedback.

'Just remember, Robbie, we are here to help people. Not to judge them. Not to fix them. Not to argue with them, but to simply help them.' He then accentuated his advice by spelling out the word. 'H E L P'

'That is our primary role, and that should always be uppermost in your thoughts when a client asks for help. OK?'

'Got it. Thanks'.

We had a busy day ahead of us.

Looking at the appointment book, I saw that Doug had written in a new appointment for me. I smiled at what I saw.

'That appointment you've written in for me. Is that a joke? Mary? Like Mary had a little lamb?'

'That's her name. Mary. She's a new client and has recently moved to the area. I met her at uni. She was going out with a friend of mine. I have not seen her for years,' he said.

'And she has two young lambs. They were born a few days ago, and she wants them castrated. I should do it because I haven't seen her for years, but I have to preg-test cows for Don Cosgrove this morning. Therefore, you get to do Mary. Have you castrated lambs before?'

I paused before answering, 'Sort of...'

'Sort of?'

'At school. We had to castrate lambs... the old way.'

'School? Castrating lambs? The old way? Robbie. Intriguing.'

'You probably don't know, but I went to an agricultural training school, which originally had been for the sons of farmers, and one day we were lining up to castrate lambs using a Luck knife, and...our teeth.'

'Some school. Sounds brutal!'

'Yes, you could say brutal... at times. This part was. The teacher showed us how to do it. The lamb was held on its back, legs in the air, exposing the scrotum. He then made a quick cut to the scrotum with the Luck knife and, applying pressure, popped both testicles through the cut. He then grabbed each testicle with his teeth and, with a sudden sideways head movement, dislodged the testicle and spat each out into a bucket. He said that it was more hygienic that way...for the lamb.'

'And you had to do that? At school?' he said with incredulity.

Snippets of a Vet's Life

'Yep. But when it was my turn...well... I fainted. So I haven't really castrated lambs before.'

'Got it. Don't get alarmed. We have an elastrator, and no teeth required!'

Doug showed me first how to apply the green rubber ring to the prong ends, and then, while one hand applies pressure to the handle, how to expand the ring.

'Once expanded, you can place the rubber ring over the base of the scrotum, release the pressure, and dislodge the ends, and the ring stays in place. Got it?'

'Got it. Much less traumatic than the old way,' I commented.

'For both you and the lambs.'

He walked toward the door, and just as he was about to leave, looked back at me and said, 'I suspect that you have never met anybody like Mary before. You might say, at university she had a reputation...,' and then, with a slight knowing smile, he turned and left.

Mary Cohurn lived on five acres near the clinic. She was about forty and seemed pleasant enough when I introduced myself.

'I was expecting my old friend Doug,' she said sharply when I introduced myself.

'Something came up suddenly, and he couldn't make it, so he sent me. OK?'

While I was getting my gear together, I tried to chat. Mary seemed a bit cold, so perhaps she was upset that Doug had passed her over to me.

'How's your day been so far?' was a standard introduction question I learned from my mentor to use with clients. Doug was naturally gregarious, whereas I was not. It was a skill that I was learning.

'OK. But I had a late night at work. Will this take much time?' she asked, suggesting by her manner that I just get on with the task.

As we walked around the side of her house and towards a pen, I continued, 'Late night. Oh.' I then asked, 'What do you do?' It was another question that Doug had taught me.

'I'm a Madam,' she said with great openness.

'Oh, that must be fun,' I said nervously.

She looked at me and raised her eyebrows as if to say, 'Fun! Are you for real?' Mary seemed immune to my attempts at being friendly.

I quietly went about the job. 'Can you help me?' and then quickly added, 'But I can do it by myself, but it would be better if you assisted.'

'Sure. Believe me, I'm not squeamish. I have seen worse than lambs' testicles!' and she laughed at her private joke.

'Now. If I can get you to hold the first lamb on his back, exposing his... testicles?'

Snippets of a Vet's Life

She did as I asked, and once the lamb was in position, I could hold the lamb's scrotum in my left hand. Using my right hand to squeeze the elastrator and expand the green rubber ring, I deftly placed the ring over the scrotum. Once in place, I released the pressure, and the rubber ring slid, effectively cutting the blood supply to the scrotum and the two testicles.

'Good. Thanks. That's it, Mary. Now the other lamb.'

She put the lamb back in the pen, and he ran off, one hind leg occasionally kicking at his belly.

I quickly attended to the other lamb.

'That's it? No antibiotics? Any aftercare?' she asked.

'No. That's all we do. I imagine they would feel a bit uncomfortable for a few days, and they may kick a bit at their belly with their hind legs, but then the scrotum shrivels up because of no blood supply, and in time the ball sack and testicles drop off.'

'I'm glad I'm not a boy lamb,' she said as though she was wincing in pain, then asked, 'Must be hard for you... doing this. Like if I were you, I think I would feel it.'

I closed down that private conversation by saying, 'Never given it a thought,' which was not the honest truth, but I felt uncomfortable talking about my testicles with Mary. I washed the elastrator under a tap, and as I was cleaning up, she asked, 'Rob. Bit of an unusual question, but can I buy some of those rubber rings?'

'Um. I'm not sure. This is my first year. What if I get Doug to call you?'

And with that, I left.

Later, when I returned to the clinic, Doug casually asked.

'So, Robbie. Were there any problems with the lamb castrations? And how was Mary?'

He had a strange smile.

'One of my friends from uni referred her to us. They were an item, and the word was that she had a bit of a reputation. I wondered how you would handle her. She was very attractive, but that was some years ago now. How's she travelling?' he said, again with a smile.

This was a side of my boss that I had not seen before. My boss, as a the young student.

'Travelling?... I know what you mean. She's travelling OK, but, she is about your age and...'

I left it at that, and then added, 'Good news! She's going to call you. But don't react. She's not complaining. For some reason, she wants to buy some of the elastrator rings. She didn't say what, and I told her she had better talk to you. OK?'

'That's a bit strange. Sure, Robbie, but what was the problem? She probably wants them for household use, such as tying the tops of large bags. I have other clients who wanted them for that purpose. In the future, if

Snippets of a Vet's Life

someone asks, it's OK to sell them some. But I'll call her. It would be good to catch up with her.'

Before I started with my next client, I had a sudden thought. I left the examination room and found Doug, who was about to make a phone call, perhaps to Mary.

'Doug...before you call, there is one thing you probably need to know about Mary. About the rubber rings she wants. It may not be very important, but she apparently works as a... Madam...somewhere in the city.' I nervously smiled.

'What! What did you say, Robbie?'

'A Madam...you know?', I repeated with a straight face. He stared at me, his face flushed. Was it anger, or perhaps was he embarrassed?

'Did I hear you say she's a Madam? Do you know what that is?'

'Sort of. But not my thing. Is it important? Like you said, she probably wants the rings for household use.'

I did all I could to restrain my face and keep a blank look.

'Household use! I bet not. Have you ever...' and he didn't finish his words.

'No. Never. I don't know a thing about all that,' and feeling my face redden with an uncomfortable blush.

'There is no way,' he repeated the words with emphasis, 'NO WAY that we are supplying her with rubber castrator rings. Imagine if the police raided them. We would end up in the paper. I can see the headline 'Coldstream Veterinary Clinic supplies brothel with rubber rings that are normally used to castrate lambs. I don't think so, Robbie! Really, why didn't you just say 'NO' when she asked? Now I have to solve the problem! Robbie! In future...think!'

'I was only trying to... help... her, as you told me, at breakfast...' I said with a calm voice and a straight face.

'Help her... HELP HER! Robbie, there is 'help' and there is 'help!' THINK about that next time,' and he stormed off.

I returned to the next client, and as I entered the room, I could not contain a slight smile.

'Now. How can I help you?'

16 – AN EVENING NEVER TO BE FORGOTTEN

'Rob, you're early. Charlotte won't be long.'

I was having second thoughts about joining the Matron and her daughter for dinner. As much as the Matron told me that Charlotte wanted to have dinner with me, I was dubious, especially after the disastrous night at the opera a few weeks earlier. I sat down, and the Matron offered me a drink.

'Scotch and Soda? Whisky? Rob?'

'Could I get something soft? I don't really drink. Perhaps Coke, if you have it?'

Opposite me on the wall, above the fireplace, was a portrait of a woman, and various photos were on the mantelpiece. They were of a young girl on a pony. I assumed that they were Charlotte. I recalled that one of the horses I had previously stomach-drenched for worms a few weeks earlier had been Charlotte's pride and joy.

The Matron reentered the room and handed me a drink.

'Charlotte?' I said, pointing to the photos. 'And the portrait. Is that you?'

She smiled. 'No. That is a portrait of my mother when she was about Charlotte's age. She looks like her, doesn't she? And that painting is worth a lot, by William Dobell. Do you know of him?'

'No. Haven't heard of that artist, but I can see the resemblance.'

I tried to sound interested, feigning interest as I studied the picture, and remembering Doug's advice to keep the Matron 'happy', we heard a loud demand from outside the room.

'Mother!' I recognised Charlotte's voice as the Matron hurried out of the room.

She sounded as though she was in a bad mood. Behind the closed door, muffled conversations escaped, one voice louder than the other. I heard a distinct 'No' from Charlotte. Shortly after, the Matron's emphatic 'Yes, you will' echoed, and a minute later, both entered the room.

'Hello, Charlotte. We meet again!' I smiled.

She ignored me, pulled a chair from the dining table, and sat down with a heavy slump, her long blonde hair falling forward. The Matron set about serving food and, at the same time, making idle chatter about nothing. To say that there was tension in the air would be an understatement. Charlotte sat and looked straight ahead, across the table towards the window, ignoring me. I was seated at one end, while the Matron occupied the other. The Matron continued with her nervous chatter, which mostly involved asking me questions.

'Do you like football, Rob?'

'Sort of,' which was not the complete truth.

'Great. And which team do you follow? Charlotte's a Collingwood follower.'

'I follow Richmond,' though I had little interest in Australian Rules Football. And with my answer, the Matron beamed at Charlotte as if I had said something profound.

'Charlotte and I went to the football game a while ago. It was great fun.'

'Oh. I said. 'Which match?' I turned my questioning gaze towards Charlotte in an attempt to engage her. No response.

'I forget,' replied the Matron. Silence followed.

'This is delicious beef,' I proffered to break the silence.

'Lamb.'

'Sorry. But still delicious.'

'Do you cook much, Rob?'

'No, except toast.'

And as I said this, the Matron, with a joyful, encouraging smile, again looked at her daughter as though I had said something earth-shattering. I thought I would try the direct approach with Charlotte by turning and asking her, 'Is that you on the pony?' pointing to one of the photos on the wall.

It did have an effect, but not the one I had hoped for. She turned her head towards me, looked down a bit, and slightly turned her head to indicate, 'Are you for real?'

The ever-effervescent Matron intruded with, 'Yes. That's Charlotte on Pinto.'

Eager to break the strained impasse, I asked, 'Was that one of the horses I drenched the other day?'

'Yes!' she said with unexpected excitement, directing herself to Charlotte and saying, 'You should have been there, Charlotte. He was so good with Pinto.' She seemed to forget that I had to use a twitch on Pinto to restrain him.

'He's a lovely horse. Such spirit,' I said, trying to be polite.

'I see that your glass is empty. Can I get you another Rob?'

The Matron got up and left the room.

Charlotte and I sat in silence. She stared across the table at the opposite wall, seemingly oblivious to me, and I randomly looked at the photos on the wall and tapped my fingers on the tablecloth.

Snippets of a Vet's Life

I was about to try another question when suddenly Charlotte slightly turned towards me, gave me a side-on stare and almost spat out at me the words,

'My Mother thinks the sun shines out of your...' but before she could finish, the Matron reentered the room with my drink in her hand.

'So good to see you two are getting along so well.' And she beamed her ever-present broad smile at me and then Charlotte, and then back to me. In return, I gave a strained smile, and the dinner continued in a similar vein. That was the last thing Charlotte said to me that night.

The next time I heard from her was at 3:00 a.m. a few weeks later. I picked up my bedside phone, fearing the worst when I saw the time.

'I want you to come and pick me up,' she said in a very demanding tone. And without explaining why or what had happened, she gave me the address where she was.

'Now?'

'Yes. Now. Take me home.'

'Take you... to your place?' I asked to clarify in case I had misread the situation. Hope always springs eternal in a young man's mind, but it was not to be on this occasion.

'Yes! Where else?' and the phone was slammed down in my ears.

I picked her up, and Charlotte didn't say a word during the trip back to the hospital, except for a terse 'thanks' as she got out and slammed the car door shut.

The following morning, very early, while I was still deep in sleep, my bedside telephone rang.

'Rob!' Through the fog of a disturbed slumber, I recognised the Matron's voice.

I struggled to come to my senses, as I said, 'Everything is OK? The horses?' I was in automatic vet mode.

'Yes. No, No. They are fine. No. Charlotte.... last night. I am so grateful you offered to pick her up from that party. Somebody had been rude to her, and her boyfriend was drunk. And Charlotte hates it when he is drunk. There was a fight, and anyway, she was so thankful. She really likes you, especially because her boyfriend drinks,' she paused, adding, 'Just like her father.'

'I'm glad to help. Give my regards to Charlotte. I've got to go. I'm running late for work;' I fumbled the truth slightly, and I ended the call.

Unusual mother, I reflected as I returned the phone to the side drawer and settled back into resuming my disturbed sleep.

Very strange girl, I thought, somewhat alluring and attractive, and because of that, I realised that she was way out of my league.

Snippets of a Vet's Life

17 – TEDDY AND TETANUS

Chris was a few years younger than me, and we had met running up a hill. Exercise had become a constant in my life, and running had formed a significant part of my routine.

Not long after I started work with Doug, I went for a run. It was the best way to explore the new town. I ran along the main street, then took a left at the major intersection at the end of the town and ran along the banks of a minor stream towards the local park. I was struck by how rural the area felt, even though the expanding suburbia was not that far distant. To one side of the park was a road that ended at the top of a hill. I ran up the hill, and from the top, when I looked towards the city, I could see the encroaching houses of suburbia. Like a fire lapping at the edge of a forest, the result was inevitable. One day, the town would be consumed by the expanding need for housing. I wanted to metaphorically slam a gate shut and keep the city out.

On the way down the hill, I passed another person who was running up the hill. As runners do, I nodded to him to acknowledge our shared activity.

We passed on a few occasions over the next few weeks when I was out running, and each time, a nod. One day, coming from different directions, we both arrived at the base of the hill. Instead of the usual head nod, this time, he looked at me, then up the hill, and then back at me, and said, 'Race?'

He won.

While getting my breath back, I introduced myself. Chris, I discovered, was in his last year at the local Seventh-day Adventist school and was very outgoing.

'What do you want to do when you leave?' I asked by way of conversation.

'Not sure,' was his not unexpected answer, and then he enquired, 'What do you do?'

'I'm a vet. I came here to work in the local clinic.'

'Cool, man. I have been thinking about doing that. We agist horses.'

'Do you? And do you ride?' I asked

'No. My little sister does. I play football. No time.'

'OK. I'm on duty, so I'd better be heading back. See you, Chris, and perhaps next time, I'll win!' But I never did.

About two months later, one Friday night, I returned from a quick run and saw the answering machine flashing. I replayed the message.

Snippets of a Vet's Life

'Hi, Rob. It's Chris. We met out running a while ago. Sorry to disturb you, but can you give me a call?' He left a phone number.

'Thanks for getting back to me. Dad's worried about one of the agister's ponies. We've tried contacting our usual vet, but the phone just rings out. I told Dad about you, and he said to give you a ring. That, OK?'

'Yes. No problem, Chris. What's the pony doing?'

'He went through a fence a few days ago. Nothing serious, just a small wound.'

'OK. Does it need stitching?'

'Yeah, maybe, but that's not the problem. Dad thinks he's now constipated, because he's kicking a bit at his stomach.'

'Oh. It's unlikely that he's constipated, but if it's colic, I'd better come and see him.'

'Dad's pretty sure he is constipated because his tail sticks out. It's a bit weird. It's like he's got an onion shoved up his bum. When can you get here?'

He gave me directions. I reset the answer phone and drove to Sunny Side Drive, and at the end, I arrived at Sunny Side Agistment.

Chris greeted me and introduced me to his father, Carl. He was shorter than Chris and perhaps less welcoming. He had a serious look on his face.

'Thanks for coming, Rob. We usually get old Peter out, but I haven't been able to contact him. He may be having one of his sick spells. Come this way.' He led me into a small shed, and as we entered, he switched on a light.

There was a sudden movement in the stall. I looked at the pony. I could see why Carl had thought the pony was constipated. It did have its tail out, as Chris had described, but it also had a stiff arch in its neck and was a bit stiff in its legs. Within seconds, the overall stiffness relaxed, but not the tail. And, as Chris had also related, there was a small gash on the pony's chest; around it, the hair was stained with black oil. There was a faint smell of tar in the air.

'How long has the pony been like this?' I asked.

'Just today. He was OK yesterday. Perhaps a bit sore after going through the fence on Monday. Sprinkles always tries to escape, so we didn't think much of it. That's how he got that gash on his chest.'

I felt a sense of dread upon hearing this information.

I clapped my hands near his head and saw what I feared: the sudden movement of the third eyelids across his eyes, then back again into the corner of each eye. I repeated the clap and observed the same result. I then firmly slapped him on his neck, and he went into the general spasm that we had observed after disturbing him by turning on the light.

Snippets of a Vet's Life

'Well, I am sorry to say, I think...in fact,' and remembering what Doug had advised always to use clear words when delivering a diagnosis, 'In fact, I am certain, Sprinkles has tetanus.'

Chris's usual happy smile left and was replaced by a look of concern. Carl responded by putting his hand up to his brow and wiping it with a handkerchief.

'Tetanus! Are you sure?'

'I've never had a case before, but the stiffness in response to touch, the third eyelid flicking across his eyes in response to a clap, yep. I can't think of any other diagnosis,' I said confidently.

'We didn't call the vet this time, when he went through the fence, because he seemed OK, so I just put some tar oil on the wound to sterilise it. I'm a great believer in tar oil, Rob. Have you ever used it?'

'I have not had any experience with tar oil, Carl,' mentally discounting the recommendation. I then asked, 'Do you know if he has ever had a tetanus shot?'

'No. Our regular vet had wanted to give him one on a few occasions when he had gone through fences, but his owner wouldn't allow it,' Carl replied.

'Why not?' I asked somewhat incredulously.

'They are Jehovah's Witnesses,' he said, as though that announcement alone was sufficient explanation.

'I don't really understand. How does that affect giving Sprinkles a tetanus shot?'

'The anti-tetanus shot is made from the blood of Clydesdale horses, and any blood-made treatment is not allowed,' he explained.

Perhaps it was my youth or inexperience; maybe I just did not think, but I said, 'Isn't that a bit silly!'

'Not to them. That's what they believe, and we respect other people's beliefs in this household,' he said in a slightly admonishing tone.

'I'm sorry. Yes, of course. It was wrong of me. But Sprinkles, let me ask, when did you first notice his tail was out?'

'About two days ago,' Carl answered.

'Why do you ask, Rob?' Chris interjected.

'Well, as I said, this is the first time I have seen tetanus, but from what I know, the longer it takes for the signs to develop, the better the chances that Sprinkle will survive.'

'So, Rob, he can survive?' Carl asked.

'Maybe. It depends on what happens over the next few days. If he goes down, then that may be the end. But what I want to do now is give him a Valium injection into his jugular vein to relax his muscles and relieve the spasms. If it's OK with you, I want to get my boss out here to have a look, just to make sure.'

'So, it may not be tetanus, you're not sure?' asked Carl.

Snippets of a Vet's Life

'I'm sure, but I want his advice on how to manage Sprinkles. Or...if you wish, we could put him down. Does the owner know?'

'No. She's away, on holiday, overseas. We can't easily contact her. So he's in our care. It's a hard call to put him down. Not that I doubt you, but its just that I wonder what Peter...' Carl once again wiped his brow.

'I get that. Happy to talk to your usual vet. But we may have to put him down. If I remember correctly, about eighty per cent of horses die or are put down if they get tetanus. That's why they should all be vaccinated.'

About an hour later, Doug joined us and confirmed my diagnosis. 'The best thing for the pony is euthanasia,' was his pronouncement.

'Before you came, Doug, Rob was telling us that about twenty per cent of horses survive with treatment,' Chris reported as though I had given them hope.

Doug looked at me with a querulous look. ' I've never had one survive. I've seen a few cases, one other horse, and a few cows. The only case I've had that survived was a dog, which took a lot of work and care.'

Chris interrupted him, 'We don't mind doing the work!'

And I added, 'I'm willing to give it a go, Doug.'

'OK. I hear what you are saying, but in the end...'

And we all knew what remained unsaid.

After Doug left, I put the plan into place. I would return later that night to give him more Valium, which hopefully would take him through the night without spasms, and Chris volunteered to sleep on a stretcher in the stable.

'And remember, any sudden moves or sounds, even the light going on, can trigger spasms, so keep everything low-key.'

'Got it. Let's pray that he survives,' and I was surprised by his reference to the Almighty.

Later that night, I returned and gave Sprinkles an injection of Valium. Even though I moved gently, approaching him caused him to go into a minor spasm; his tail went out, his ears were erect, and he arched his neck. I waited, and it passed, and I injected the drug.

His response to the treatment earlier in the day had been quick. He had noticeably relaxed to the point where he could start eating chaff from his feeder.

This time, the response was slower. I clapped my hands, and there was a flickering across his corneas of the third eye.

I gave him more, and after this dose, he noticeably relaxed and swayed slightly.

'Careful, he just may go down. Valium can do that. We will have to be careful with the dosage. Getting the balance may be a problem.'

'What happens if he goes down?' he asked.

Snippets of a Vet's Life

'We will have to lift him onto his feet physically. And it will take more than you, me, and your father to do it, even though he is a Welsh Mountain pony. While I was home, I looked up tetanus in my vet notes. If a horse goes down, it tries to get up, which stimulates a massive and general spasm, and apparently, it goes stiff in the legs. Unassisted, Sprinkles will not be able to get up by himself.'

'It will just be me and you in the morning, if that's OK. Dad's strict about the Sabbath. We fought over it after you left. I'm beginning to think it is all crap, but Adventists believe in the sanctity of the seventh day of the week, and that is Saturday. We go by the Hebrew calendar, where Saturday is the Sabbath.'

I came from a family with strong religious beliefs, on my mother's side, but this was on a whole new level. When my middle brother was a teenager, he wanted to play baseball on a Sunday team, but my mother prohibited it in observance of the Lord's Day. I occasionally wondered what my brother thought of my father allowing and even encouraging me to attend the local pony club each Sunday morning. It was a rare example of my parents disagreeing on parenting issues.

'Well, as you said earlier, perhaps we should pray … for Sprinkles, ' I said with a slight hesitation, hiding a slight discomfort, then left.

I was not surprised when the phone rang at 7:00 am the following day.

'Sprinkles is on the ground.'

My boss had said, 'I would put him down, Robbie. He's only going to suffer. Apparently, people who come down with tetanus suffer extreme muscle spasms that can fracture bones. So, the kindest thing to do is to put him out of his misery.'

When I arrived, four boys about Chris's age greeted me, but none were as tall.

He had a smile once again on his face as he said, 'I called on some mates. Enough?'

'Great! Now, don't forget. No sudden noises or movements. Even though Sprinkles is on the ground, he can still hurt himself trying to get up, and he can also hurt you, so be ready to jump out of the way if he struggles. Now, Chris, your job is to control his head and neck. He will try to throw it back to get up, so it's your job to control him. Make sure he doesn't hit you in the face. OK. The first thing I will do is give him a shot of Valium to relax him. Then, on three, let's all lift together. Slowly and follow my lead.'

Due to our efforts, he again experienced a general spasm, including one in his chest, which prevented him from breathing.

'Ok. Good. Up. Keep pushing,' and our combined efforts placed him upright. I was relieved when he relaxed a little, was able to stand, and more importantly, take a breath.

'Now. Everybody. Just stay where you are. Chris, if possible, keep his head facing forward. I'm hoping that he will just relax and hold his weight, and then when that happens, gradually remove your hands, boys. But be ready; he might just go stiff again and fall.'

But he did not fall. While we held him in an upright position, he relaxed a bit and was able to take another breath. His stiff legs relaxed, and he took his weight, and the boys could step back.

'Praise the Lord,' said someone.

'Maybe, but your efforts helped the Lord a lot!'

Chris had a big smile on his face. 'That was fantastic. How did you know what to do if this is your first tetanus case?' he asked me.

'I just do know it,' was my lame response, and then, after a few seconds of thought, I said, 'However, I spent the last two years of my vet studies assisting in large animal surgery, and that mainly involved removing bone chips from racehorses' knees, or colic surgery, and removing parts of damaged intestines. And then, after surgery, the tricky part happened. Getting a partially awake horse on its feet.'

'Using pulleys?' one of them suggested.

'No. The trick is holding them down for as long as possible in the recovery stall, a special, enclosed stall lined with rubber. The door is also lined with rubber. But just like us, coming out of a long anaesthetic is a slow process, and that's why we are in bed when we wake up. So, we don't try to walk before the anaesthetic drugs have worn off, and perhaps fall, and hurt ourselves.'

'It sounds dangerous,' one boy said, and another, 'Sounds like fun!'

'It is dangerous, being in that stall, and that is what the students do on the surgery roster that day. They hold the horse down on the ground by laying on its neck until enough of the anaesthetic drug has worn off so that the horse can get up and regain its balance on the first attempt.'

'Wow,' was one response. 'I want to be a vet,' another said enthusiastically.

'Occasionally, a horse tries to get up before it is ready, and they crash down, and unfortunately, they can break a leg, and then there is nothing else that can be done except end its life.'

'Why can't you just fix their leg, like in people?' Chris asked.

'Well. We can usually fix the break. Like in dogs and cats. But horses, cows…but then there is a problem. So, what is it?'

There was a prolonged silence, broken by an excited, 'I know! I've got it. You can't get them up again?'

Snippets of a Vet's Life

'Correct. Often, after the surgery to fix the break, which can only be done under anaesthesia with the horse on the ground, when the horse tries to get up, during recovery, the weight of the horse itself breaks the cast that has been placed on the broken leg. Thus, the injured bone re-breaks. So, you end up with a mess, and the horse has to be put down.'

While I was talking, I watched Sprinkles. He seemed stable on his legs and quietly nudged his food, but he could not eat even though he tried. I felt his masseter muscles, the large muscles on either side of his jaw and below his eyes, which, when working, moved his jaw side to side while he ate. However, his jaw muscles were tight, and I wasn't surprised that he could not take a bite. In people, the old name for tetanus was 'Lockjaw', and for good reason, because that is precisely what happens to their jaw due to the circulating toxin.

The boys were enthusiastic learners, so I was not surprised when one of them asked, 'What causes tetanus? Is it something we catch?'

For that knowledge, I was indebted to a great teacher, Dr. Woolcock, who taught microbiology to second-year veterinary students. It was only when I reread the notes I had made at the start of his lecture series that I finally got an insight into what he was teaching. There was an ongoing war inside each of us. It was only when the bad guys, the bugs or the infectious agents that cause disease, got the upper hand that we saw disease. Most of the time, the body's troops, as he called them, could keep the baddies at bay, but sometimes, the bad guys got the upper hand, won the war, and took over. Tetanus was a good example.

I liked having an audience, and I was about to talk about what caused tetanus when I suddenly remembered: the clinic opened at 9:00 am, and I was on duty.

Five days later, the boys, all now looking tired after many interventions, walked the now recovered Sprinkle out of the stable and into the paddock. They all had a look of achievement on their faces.

'Praise the Lord,' Chris said as he shook my hand, and then added, 'and the vet!'

18 – GETTING DOWN TO BUSINESS

About a month later, my contract with Doug came to an end, and a new graduate was going to take my place. Doug had been a good mentor, and working with him had been a good first job. I did not realise at the time that this was the last time I worked for another vet.

When I left the Coldstream Veterinary Clinic, I had no plan except for some vague thought that I would need to find a new job, which would require me to move. I thanked Doug for all that he had done for me, said goodbye to Samantha, who surprisingly gave me a hug, before I walked down the stairs and went home to the Green Cottage.

I was surprised that I was not alarmed at the prospect of not having a job. I was unsure what I would do, but I wasn't worried, which I thought was unusual, as I later drifted off to sleep.

I was dreaming, and a phone rang. I was confused. Where was the phone? I couldn't locate it, which was stressing me. The phone had come to dominate my life, and my weekends had often been determined by being always available on the phone. In the dream, I was running and then falling, but I still could not find the phone. Confusion. Panic! And then I woke up, sweating.

'Hello,' I said, attempting to get to my senses, but I was not quite awake and still amid the dream.

'Oh, Good. Rob. You're there. Jane here.'

'Hi, Jane. How can I help you?' I said, recognising her voice.

'I've got a mare with colic. Remember Dorothy? She's not getting any better.'

I remembered Dorothy with affection. She was the first mare I had pregnancy tested, and she was also the mare that had nearly finished my career as a vet when she attempted to kick me in the head on my first visit to Jane's property.

Now wide awake, I said,' That's no good, Jane, but I should let you know that I don't work for Doug any more, and you should give him a call.'

'I did. And there was no answer. So I've called you. Can you help? She's in a bad way'

I considered her request. She was Doug's client, and now that I was not working for the clinic, I should not have any professional contact with her. The ethics of the profession were clear and straightforward. But she had reached out for help. Jane didn't know about ethics, but she needed my help. Her pony needed attention. And

Doug had always told me that our role, as vets, was to help people, so I said,

'I'll be there as quickly as possible,' I said, confident I was doing the 'right thing'.

'But Jane, all I have is a stomach tube and a stethoscope and some paraffin oil, but no drugs. I left them at the clinic when I departed. But I'll see what I can do. To help you. We may just have to call Doug if I need any drugs.

Once again, it was a lonely car trip in the dead of night with only a few others on the road. I had time to reflect that, in a way, it was fitting for me to be driving to Jane's. She and Sonia had been the first farm call I attended as a newly minted vet. And even more fitting was that it was the same mare I had seen that first day, the mare that had tired to kick me as I pregnancy tested her.

Luckily, the colic resolved about an hour after administering paraffin oil through a stomach tube.

They were interested in what had happened, and why I wasn't working for Doug anymore, but I mildly dismissed them with the words, 'Things just happen. I came to the end of the contract.'

'What are your plans, Rob?' Sonia asked as I was about to leave.

'I don't have any,' I replied. 'I guess I will have to get a job somewhere.'

'But that will mean that you'll leave the area and that's a shame, Rob,' Jane said. 'You're good with horses, and we need a good horse vet around here. Doug's not that interested.'

'I'm sure he will work something out. He's got a new guy coming in to help him. So, good night,' I said.

I drove back to the Green Cottage and returned to my sleep.

About lunchtime the following day, the phone rang.

'Hi Rob. It's Beth. We met once, at Jane's. I've got this racehorse who is agisted with us, and it has been lame for a while. The owner has had a few city vets come here to examine him, but nobody has been able to fix him. And Jane said you were good with horses, and to give you a call. The owner is a bit desperate.'

I was still concerned about ethics. Beth was not strictly a client of Doug's practice. She owned and operated an agistment property with her husband, Edmond. On one occasion, I had to stitch up one of her client horses while it was under the care of Jane Miller. However, she usually used the city vets, mainly because Beth and her husband agisted racehorses, and the owners usually had their preferred veterinarians.

But, as it transpired, that call started the next stage of my career. I became a horse vet, working out of the Green Cottage.

Word travelled, and I was off and running in my

practice, all thanks to Jane Miller and me doing the 'right thing'. Admittedly, it was not a conventional practice with a clinic, staff, and a physical 'presence.' In fact, I worked out of the boot of my car. It was a horse practice that relied on 'word of mouth.' And word of me was spreading, which was excellent for my young ego.

But there was one problem. Ethically, I should not have done it. I was operating in Doug's area, and I had worked for Doug. I countered my argument by knowing that Doug didn't particularly like doing horse work, but deep down, I realised it was not the right thing to do.

And quickly the business grew, and the workload increased. But I had no training in business, and problems with money started to occur.

Some families have a tradition of business ownership, and as children, the necessary skills become ingrained in their psyche.

But I was the 'scion' of working-class folk. My grandparents once owned a market-garden allotment and worked for themselves, but they lost everything in the Great Depression of the 1930s. From then on, my mother's father worked the land as an employee. My grandfather on my father's side was a postie and delivered letters twice daily throughout his working life. And for all their working lives, my parents were employed.

Such is the roll of the dice at birth. As I entered the bank in Seville, I set aside my mental reflections. I had an appointment to see the bank manager, Robert Goodfellow.

'Take a seat,' Robert said as I entered his small office.

I sat silently as he read some sheets from a file... my file.

In my fourth year at university, I was living in Kendall Hall, the residence for the fourth and fifth year Veterinary Students at Werribee, about an hour's drive from the city. I quickly formed the opinion that I needed a more reliable car than the clapped-out student car that had served me well when I lived in Trinity College, which is attached to the main campus of the University of Melbourne.

But how did I fund a car purchase when I was a student?

I sought help from my older brother, then a young accountant, who assisted me in establishing an account with the bank and securing a loan. As a student, I managed to keep up with the monthly repayments.

'OK, Rob. You have a good record with the bank, so how can I help you?'

I explained that I had recently started my own veterinary practice and operated from home. I had formed the opinion that I needed an overdraft to help me manage my creditor's payments while waiting for clients to settle their accounts with me.

Snippets of a Vet's Life

'While waiting for your client's money to flow in, your money continues to flow out of your account as you pay bills, and if too much flows out, you have a cash flow problem'

'Yes. That is the problem, I think. When I started, I had savings in my account. However, I have noticed that as I'm getting busier, I'm now running low on funds, and lately, I haven't always been able to pay the bills on time. I was wondering if the bank could help me?'

'Of course we can. That's what I'm here for. To help you in your business. What you need is an overdraft. But first, a few questions.'

He seemed satisfied, and about ten minutes later, after answering a few more questions, I left the bank with a new business chequebook, a $5000 overdraft, and some advice.

'Don't let it go over the limit, Rob, or you will find that I will be calling you on a Monday morning to find out why you are over?'

And a few weeks later, one Monday morning, my phone rang.

'I'm sorry to disturb you, but your overdraft has been overdrawn for a few days. I'm wondering when you can bring it back into order.'

'Oh, sorry!' I said, feeling embarrassed. 'I have some cheques lying around, so I will pay them into my account today. Is that OK?'

'Yes, that will be fine. And Rob, if I can offer you some advice, I would suggest getting into the habit of regularly depositing your cheques into your account, or getting some help around the office.'

And that is why, a few weeks later, I gave Joan Philpott, a semi-retired bookkeeper, a job. She always answered, 'Yes, dear,' whenever I suggested a change in how we handled outstanding accounts or, for that matter, in how we ran the business.

Before joining me, having children, and moving to the Yarra Valley, Joan worked for a while in the accounts payable department of a large city share broking firm.

The following Monday morning, the bank manager was on the phone again: the overdraft was 'over.' I told him about Joan, and he seemed somewhat placated.

Cash flow continued to be a problem, and apart from the inherent fact that many of our clients could not afford horses, but they did not know that they could not afford them, there was an inherent problem with how we managed our outstanding accounts.

'Joan, I have thought about the accounts. If we send out the statements at the start of the month instead of the middle of the month, they may pay us a bit quicker. So next month, can you send out the statements at the start of the month?'

'Yes, dear, ' and she continued whatever she was doing.

Snippets of a Vet's Life

I had concluded that whenever Joan said, 'Yes, dear,' it usually meant, 'No, dear.'

I followed her response, asking, 'So…is that a Yes?'

Silence ensured, so I was not hopeful about the outcome.

'Joan, not wanting to be rude or disrespectful, but do you think calling me 'dear' is the right thing to say, considering that you…well…to be slightly blunt…that you work for me?'

I was not very assertive at this stage of my career and lacked skills in managing employees.

'Yes, dear,' was her response. She turned away and ended the conversation, and the topic was never addressed again.

She was to work for me for the next twenty years. In time 'Yes dear' was replaced, with 'Yes Boss,' but not always.

Rod Graham

19 – A ROOSTER, A DONKEY, AND A PAIR OF SPEEDOS

'Please come in,' I said to my unexpected but most welcome visitor at the back door. I had earlier arrived home after a morning horse call, and even though there was a chill in the air, I was about to leave for a swim when there was a soft knock at the back door.

'I'm sorry to disturb you, Dr McBride, but I have a problem with Percival, my rooster,' my landlady explained as she entered the Green Cottage carrying a cage.

'He's suddenly lost his voice!' she said in some alarm. We always addressed each other in very formal terms. I was Dr McBride, never Rob, except on one occasion, and she was always Mrs Pridham, never Pamela or Pammy, as Jimmy Dunne called his lifelong friend.

I directed her to the sitting room, and I was thankful I had lit a fire earlier in the day to ward off the unseasonable cold temperature.

'Would you like a cup of tea or coffee?' I asked as she sat down.

Snippets of a Vet's Life

'Yes, tea, thank you. That is so kind of you,' she said with a precise, slightly clipped English accent. I left the room, but as I was about to turn on the kettle, I heard her gasp as though in fright.

Before I could investigate, Mrs Pridham rushed out of the sitting room, clutching Percival's cage under her arm.

'I'm sorry. I must go,' she said, quickly moving past me, opening the kitchen door, and leaving.

'Have I upset you?' I called out to my retreating landlady. 'And what about Percival?' But there was no response.

I returned to the sitting room, perplexed. The windows were closed, and a fire quietly burned in the fireplace. There was nothing out of place. Her sudden exit was unexplained, but it was somewhat fortunate because I remembered little of my lectures on the diseases and ailments of chickens or, for that matter, birds in general. The reason for her sudden exit was a complete mystery to me. But as so often was the case, the phone interrupted things.

'Is that... the vet?' a woman asked, unsure of her words.

'Oh, Good. You...you don't know me, but a friend, Jane Miller, recommended you a few days ago.' She continued in a rushed, nervous voice, almost running out of breath and ignoring my question, 'I have a major problem, and I can't get to my regular vet! I hope you can help me. I need a vet now! My donkey is in my pool, and I can't get...get her out. Can you help me?'

'Is her head above water? Is she drowning? Is there somebody with you who could help?' I asked with alarm.

'No. She is OK. She's not drowning. Her head is above water, but I am worried that she is distressed. And there is nobody to help me. My husband is at work, and I am also worried about his response. Can you come now?'

About 10 minutes later, I turned into her driveway, which led me up a short incline and delivered me behind a house. I parked and immediately saw the problem: a donkey quietly standing in a medium-sized pool.

'Thanks for coming so quickly. I am worried. I'm April, and she is Peaches. I'm not sure how this happened. I went...went out for about half an hour, and when...when I returned, I found Peaches in the pool.... I tried my normal vet, but there was no answer, so I called you. Can you get her out?'

And a light rain started falling.

'I'll give it a go. Luckily, I swim most days, so I have my Speedos in the car. So if you can show me where I can change, I'll be able to jump in the pool and make sure she is OK.'

Five minutes later, I lowered myself gently into the cold water and gradually approached Peaches. She turned her head, gave a hew-haw as though in welcome, and remained standing in the same position, but her eyes never left me, as though she viewed me with distrust. She wore a halter, and I attached a rope, gently pulling on it to see if she would respond. However, she did not move. Donkeys can resist movement if they choose not to. For reasons I did not understand, standing in the pool's shallow end, with her head, neck, and rump above the water, seemed to be where she wanted to be.

'She can be a bit stubborn,' her owner said, offering encouragement and an apology for Peaches' reluctance to move.

'That's OK.' I shivered.

I checked her out as best I could. She stood on four legs, so nothing was broken. Her pupils appeared to be the same on both sides, and both reacted when I quickly moved my hand toward each eye, so she was unlikely to have a head injury. 'No sign of concussion,' I said.

'How are you going to get her out?' April asked, as if I had a ready solution.

'Not sure, but I will think of something. Can you get some of her favourite food? I want to see if she is motivated by food.'

A few minutes later, April returned with a bucket. As she handed it to me, I could smell the alluring aroma. I held out the bucket just in front of Peaches's head. She reached forward and greedily started eating molasses-enriched oats.

'That's great! It gives us a chance. At least we can get her to move now,' I observed as I shivered in the cold water. The rain was getting heavier, but April did not seem worried.

'You should get out of the rain. No use in both of us getting wet,' I said through chattering teeth. It was cold!

'I'm good. We ski a lot, and it can be much worse than this. Can I do anything to help?'

'Not sure. Do you have a ramp or something similar to that?'

'A ramp? I'll check. My husband has a lot of things in his shed. I'll be back in a minute.'

While I waited, I removed the bucket from near in front of Peaches, and while pulling gently on the lead rope, I got the donkey to follow me and the bucket of food.

I learned a few years earlier, that taking time to look about the local environment for resources is always a good strategy.

As a new vet student, the class had a lecture on emergency care and CPR, or more correctly cardio-pulmonary resuscitation, in the first week of lectures. Then, as fate would have it, as a new friend, Nigel, and I were eating lunch that day, a man collapsed in front of us. The friend and I looked at each other, almost with a look of joy that here was a situation where we could apply our newly acquired information. While he did CPR, I did mouth-to-mouth. Unfortunately, the unconscious man, whom we later discovered was the Professor of Chemistry, had eaten before the debilitating event, and probably in response to Nigel's, perhaps over-enthusiastic chest compression, as I was to push another breath into the Professor, he vomited tuna into my open mouth. I stood up and gagged, stopped mouth-to-mouth, and helped with the chest compression. However, it was clear after a few minutes that our efforts were unsuccessful, and he was not breathing. At about this stage, the ambulance arrived, and they took over his care. But within a few minutes, they pronounced him dead. I stood up, and we both moved away as the body was lifted and put on a stretcher and taken towards the ambulance parked on a nearby road. And then, as I watched, I noticed the swimming pool that was on the other side of the road.

'Rob,' I said to Nigel. 'The swimming pool! There would have been a resuscitation unit for sure in there!'

If we had taken the time at the start of the emergency to assess the available resources, the unfortunate professor's outcome may have been different.

It was a lesson I have never forgotten, so, approaching Peaches, I looked around to see what was available to help me get her out of the pool. A metal ladder was attached to the pool's sides at both ends. It's great for people to get out, but not very useful if you have four legs. What I needed was a ramp.

'Any luck?' I asked expectantly as April returned

'No. I'm sorry. What now? I'm worried that my husband will return soon from work. He doesn't like the donkeys at the best of times, and he is passionate about the pool and keeping it clean.' And as she spoke, we scanned the pool.

'First, we must get Peaches out; then we can worry about the pool and your husband. OK?'

'Sorry. It's just that he can get VERY upset.'

I shivered as I listened to her concerns and unconsciously looked about, observing a bale of hay leaning against a nearby wall. I had a sudden brainwave. 'Do you have any other bales of hay nearby?'

'Yes. In the shed. Do you want to feed her hay? She seems very happy with the molasses…'

'I need about six, perhaps seven bales. Show me where they are, will you?'

I climbed out of the pool and shivered as the wind hit me. A few minutes later, I returned with two bales, one in each hand. The effort warmed me up, but the slight relief was short-lived. I threw both bales into the pool and jumped back in. As I had hoped, the floating bales gradually became sodden with pool water and sank to the bottom.

'Great. This is going to work,' I said as I clambered out of the pool.

I collected more hay bales and threw them into the pool. I then reluctantly jumped back in and, with some effort, manoeuvred the sodden bales towards the shallow end. Luckily, even though they were now underwater, I could move them and create a hay bale staircase out of the pool.

'You are so clever,' April said with enthusiasm. I agreed cheekily with a smile. I was feeling chuffed with myself.

After I finished my construction, I used the bucket of food to position Peaches at the underwater base of the staircase. With a bit of encouragement, she clambered up the stairs and soon stood on the lawn. She put her head down and, ever the opportunist, started eating the lawn like nothing had happened.

April had a broad smile on her face. 'Thank you. Thank you.' And then, after a few seconds, a slightly worried look crossed her face. 'The bales...? Can you get them out? My husband will be so angry.'

I stood on the pool edge and shivered, then sighed at her request and jumped back into the freezing pool. Few people know this, but throwing dry hay bales into a pool is more straightforward than removing water-laden hay bales, from a pool.

About 25 minutes later, I rolled the last bale onto the pool's edge. After allowing the water to drain, which took about 5 minutes, I returned the last bale to the shed as I had done with the previous bales. The surface of the pool was littered with bits of straw. My teeth chattered as I asked for a towel.

I'm so grateful, Rob. I can clean up the rest. You'd best be off because my husband, Bruce, will be home soon,' she paused and smiled. 'I'm not sure how to explain to him why a young man, to him a stranger, dressed only in Speedos and shivering and blue with the cold, is standing near our pool on a very wet autumn day.'

She stopped as if considering what to say, 'I would have to come clean about Peaches in the pool, and that would really upset him.'

'I agree. It does look … odd, so I'd best be off then.' I started walking toward my car, shivering but wrapped in the towel. Then I turned back toward her and said, as if it were a mere afterthought, 'I can send you an invoice… OK?'

Like many young vets, I was still uncomfortable asking for money, especially for myself. Not surprisingly, I now had no desire to go for my regular swim, so I returned to the Green Cottage and stocked up the waning fire. As I sat, I reconsidered my earlier encounter with my landlady. What troubled me was Mrs Pridham's sudden exit. But as much as I thought and looked out the window, it was a mystery, but as I found out, not for long.

Two days later, I received a letter from Mrs Pridham.

'Dear Dr McBride, please excuse my sudden exit the other day. When I sat in the sitting room and looked around, I saw an old hunting print on the wall. As I looked closer, I was stunned, and there is no other word for how I reacted to what I saw. The lady sitting on the horse was somebody I vaguely knew, from my childhood in London. The memory stirred a need in me to find out more. I looked up Debrett's, which you may not know, lists all those in the peerage, and found her and her husband. And I found this information:

"Albert Brassey, Master of the Heythrop, and his wife, the Hon Matilda, and their London address was 29 Berkeley Square."

And that address... stirred a further memory. It was the last private house in Berkeley Square. I was out walking one morning with my grandmother, and I remember visiting one of her closest friends. My memory of her face is blurred, but I knew that she was a lady of great character. She is the lady in your print called the 'Heythrop Hunt.' Also listed was their country address: Heythrop, Chipping Norton. And by coincidence, when my late husband and I married, we spent part of our honeymoon in the house in the print's background. So, please forgive my rude leaving, and *you will be pleased to know that Percival is regaining his voice!*

Pamela Pridham.'

The mystery was solved.

I looked closer at the old hunting print on my sitting room wall. I had purchased it a few weeks earlier, as a XMAS present for myself, from The Old London Print Shop in Hawthorn. It was titled 'The Heythrop Hunt' and depicted a man sitting comfortably astride his chestnut hunter. Slightly behind and to one side of him was a woman dressed in dark riding clothes, sitting in a side-saddle. Both were ready for the hunt. And to the back of them, in a lesser role, was a man, also astride a horse, perhaps a servant, and dressed in the livery of the hunt, in control of a pack of foxhounds, and a terrier. And in the far distance, a single-story grand manor house.

I looked closer at the print's date: 1896.

I was amazed. Mrs Pridham had some vague recollection of the young woman in print. She then mentally aged the image of the woman and realised she had met her in the 1920s, when my landlady was a child and out for a walk one day in Grosvenor Square, London, with her grandmother.

I was also thankful that Percival was regaining his voice. Mrs Pridham's sudden exit two days earlier gave me time to review my lecture notes on birds, and there was a slightly quirky note about how some roosters can get laryngitis from too much crowing.

One mystery was solved, but how or why Peaches came to be in the swimming pool remained unsolved. However, a few weeks later, I saw April in the local supermarket.

'Peaches is great, back to normal. And once again, thank you. I've told my donkey friends all about you.'

'That is good of you. Did your husband ever find out?'

'No. But he was perplexed by the amount of straw he found in the pool filter the following weekend when he was cleaning the pool.'

'Will you ever tell him?

'Maybe. Perhaps, one day,' she paused before continuing with a cheeky smile, 'He can be a bit of an ass when it comes to his pool'.

20 – THANK YOU FOR YOUR SERVICE, MAX

It was a new day, but I felt off-colour and stayed in bed, the kind of unwell that dulls the edges of thought.

Fortunately, or perhaps unfortunately, depending on the state of my bank account, the phone remained silent, and I drifted in and out of sleep. When it finally rang around 6:30 pm., the migraine had lifted, but left that hollow, delicate feeling behind. I felt like I'd been washed out and pegged on the line.

'Yes?' I answered, my voice barely convincing.

This was a new challenge, balancing illness and professional responsibility. When I was employed, a sick day was simply managed by making a phone call to the clinic, and leaving me with a clear conscience. But now, running my own practice, I had to weigh my own well-being against the needs of others. It hit me early on: clients don't care if you're sick, not unkindly, just practically. They have animals that need help, my help. That pressure of pushing through when I should be recovering nudged something deeper, a familiar anxiety I thought I'd left in my teenage years.

'Rob? Is that you? You don't sound too flash. Max McClintock here.'

I had met Max at the local Quarter Horse Club a few weeks earlier. The club's secretary asked me to speak to members on one of their club days, who commented, as an introduction, that I was 'flavour of the month' amongst the local horse owners.

Her comment was uplifting, and word of mouth was helping me. However, as I would learn with experience, my popularity could vary. One day, I felt like I was sitting on the right hand of God, but the next day, I was associated with the Devil.

'Good to catch you, Rob. I must say I was impressed with your talk the other day. Hence this call. You probably do not know, but my wife, Anne and I have an agistment property. I should point out that it was her idea. She gets the agistment money, and I get the added work!' he said, with humour in his voice.

'Anyway, Rob. There is this agister, and she has a slight problem with her horse.'

'A quarter horse?'

'No. We are not so lucky. It's actually a big brute of a horse. As you may have noticed, Rob, I'm new to the horse world. I think her horse is a Packeron...or something like that, and crossed with a thoroughbred.'

'Do you mean a Percheron?' I suggested.

'Yes…. whatever. But he is causing us a real headache. The owner can't control him, and now he has gone through the barbed wire fence and cut his chest, and she is freaking out. I realise that it is a bit late in the day, but can you come?'

Max's directions to his property, 'Happy Acres,' were perfect. This was not always the case when locating a new client's horse.

The wooden fence abutting the dirt road had been recently painted. As I approached, a welcoming Max stood by the open metal gates, with a paint brush in his hand.

'Hi Rob. Give us a ride to the house?'

As a way of small talk, which I was not very good at, I complimented him on his directions to his property.

'Army training, Rob,' was all he said.

'Army? Did you go to Vietnam?'

'Yep. Nasho,' he answered, referring to the shortcut, slightly derogatory name for National Service and conscription that had plagued many young men's lives in the late 1960s and early 1970s.

'I missed out on that lottery,' I added.

We drove on in silence.

My memory took me back to my student days and my brief contact with the Army Reserve.

Snippets of a Vet's Life

In 1972, Nigel Hines was a fellow vet student, and we both lived in college. It was the time of the Vietnam War, and all young men who were twenty years old were eligible for the draft.

Twice a year, the Defence Department conducted a public lottery based on the month of birth. It was a nerve-racking yet straightforward game of chance for men of the required age, and full-time students were not exempt. Twelve small, round white ceramic balls, each marked with an individual month on the outside, were placed in a large, clear plastic circular container. The handle would be turned to mix the balls, and a minor dignitary would then pull them out one by one until no more were needed, selecting a ball that indicated a specific month. If your birth-date fell in one of the selected months, you were 'in' and called up to join the Army for the next 2 years. If you 'won' the lottery but chose not to join the Army, absconded, or merely disappeared voluntarily, you were labelled a 'Draft Dodger.'

Nigel was at the top of our class. He was my intellectual elite and, at times, could be unexpectedly street-smart. And Nigel had a plan to offset the risk of getting drafted. He planned to join the Army Reserve Officers' Corps, and if accepted, any required service would be deferred until he graduated. And, he cleverly calculated that by the time he graduated, Australia would be out of the Vietnam War, and the Army would not want him. He would avoid the uncertainty of the draft process because, by default, if a person's birth month was picked and the Army Reserve Officers Corps had accepted the young man, you were exempt from spending two years in the Army and probably in Vietnam.

It was a good plan, so I followed his lead and submitted my application. But there was an unexpected outcome. Nigel was accepted, but the Army, in a very blunt letter, rejected my application on 'mental health grounds'.

Perhaps I was a bit laissez-faire in the interview with the Army's admission psychiatrist. I had told him about the panic attacks that had plagued me since my early teenage years. Whatever the reason, I was back in the Draft. Maybe I was a bit mad or did not have the mindset to lead others into combat, and which may have resulted in their death.

Unfairly, I reflected, having 'mental health' issues was a hindrance to leadership, but not to being drafted into the ranks, and possibly killing North Vietnamese soldiers, or being killed for the cause.

But I was lucky. My birth month, October, stayed firmly in the mix. It was not drawn out on draft selection day, so I could continue my studies without being drafted by the Army.

'I was in the last draft. I guess you were in one of the early ones?' I said to Max, with a touch of humour in my voice, looking straight ahead as I drove towards the house.

'Not so subtle, Rob. Yes, I was in the first, and my month came up. But the Army was good for me. It gave me the life skills I needed and taught me discipline, so you won't get an anti-army argument from me.'

'I wasn't suggesting anything. Now tell me about the horse problem...'

21 – MEETING BOS

I parked the car on the broad gravel expanse in front of the house, and Max said, 'Come this way and as a special treat, you'll meet my wife, Anne.'

'And who have we got here, Maxie?' a woman asked as we entered the kitchen. She was surprisingly well-dressed for the local area and looked slightly younger than Max.

'This is the new vet I told you about the other day. Rob...'

'Well, Robert,' she said, and from then on, she always called me Robert. 'Max has told me how impressed he was with you. And what brings you to our little acreage?'

'He's here 'cause that stupid horse owned by Melinda has run away again...I just...'

'Max, you know she's behind in her agistment payments,' Anne said, interrupting him and then turning towards me, adding, 'Maxie has his little favourites.'

'Now, Anne, I'll say something to her,' he promised in

Snippets of a Vet's Life

response.

'If you don't, I will' was Anne's final determination.

'Anyway, this time, her stupid pig-headed horse has gone through a fence and cut his chest.'

'Oh. I wondered what the screaming was about.'

'And you didn't think to look out the window?' Max playfully questioned her.

'I've been busy making your dinner, Maxie,' she said, probably for my benefit, and then continued, 'You know the deal. Managing the problems is your job, Max. I just collect the money. Has he explained that to you, Robert?'

'No, actually, he did not...'

'He always makes me out to be the kept woman, but I'm not. I see myself as more in the role of the long-suffering wife...Living out here was his idea.'

I reflected on what Max had previously told me about the arrangement, and I concluded that Max and Anne seemed to have different views on why they had an agistment property.

'Now, Anne. We don't need to go along that street. This way, Rob'.

He led me out the back door, past the in-ground pool, a well kept veggie plot surrounded by a newly trimmed hedge and a tennis court, and onto a graded internal road. In the distance, by the light of the dying day, I saw a young woman, clearly distressed and holding a baby. Tied to a post was a large chestnut horse, seemingly not distressed, attempting to graze at what he could reach by straining at the rope. As I approached them, the horse lifted his head and looked at me, perhaps judging me, then dropped his head and continued attempting to reach the grass just beyond his reach.

'Melinda, this is Rob, the new vet.'

'Hi, Rob,' she said and then continued in rapid-fire, 'Thanks for coming so quickly. He's cut his chest. Will he die? I worried about tetanus. He has been such a naughty boy. You see, he always runs away when he doesn't want to do anything. He's such a handful. Do you need my help?' she asked, looking down at the baby in her arms.

'Hold on, Melinda,' Max said. Rob has just arrived and doesn't know anything about your situation. So, just slow down. Rob, can I help you in some way?'

It was evident that Melinda was occupied with holding the baby, and I wondered if she had been attempting to lead the horse and hold the baby simultaneously.

'Thanks, Max. That would be great. First, let's untie him.'

But Max put a straining hand on my arm.

'I wouldn't do that, my young friend, without perhaps first tranquillising him. He is powerful, even for me. If he wants to, he will flick his head to the other side, pull the rope out of your hands, and run away. He does that if he doesn't want to do something.'

'I usually get him to cooperate by holding a feed bucket in front of him if I lead him anywhere, but today, with the baby...' Melinda explained.

'OK,' I said, 'No problem. Let me untie him and show you a trick to stop him from running away.'

'You're the boss, Rob,' said Max, perhaps slightly apprehensively and crossing his arms simultaneously. 'Luckily, I've closed the front gates...' with a slight smile on his face, possibly suggesting an unsaid, 'and we shall see just how smart a young fellow you are.'

'We need the feed bucket. He's going to run away, I'm telling you. Nobody can control him,' Melinda said with rising apprehension.

'We will see,' was all I said.

I untied the rope and held him securely by the halter, firmly in control of his big head, and as I did so, I formed a loop with the rope and put the loop in his mouth so that the rope passed from one side to the other of his mouth. Then, I passed the free end of the rope through the buckle underneath the halter and took up the slack. I released my hold on his head, and he went to drag the rope out of my hands with a swift movement of his head away from me. I knew his trick. I had seen it in 'naughty' Shetland ponies when they wanted to escape their owners. But this time, it did not work for him. Just as he went to run away, I drew back suddenly on the lead, and because it was through his mouth, I had the required leverage to bring his head back, facing towards me. He tried again with a sudden head flick away from me, and again, I applied sudden pressure to the rope in the opposite direction, and his head snapped back towards me.

'That's it, mate,' I said to the horse as I patted his neck, 'I'm in control. New rules.'

As I relaxed my hold on the rope, he just stood there, looking at me, and then away. I liked him. He was my type of horse: strong, with a bit of attitude, and a chestnut.

'That's amazing, Rob,' Max said, noticeably relieved and, I wondered, perhaps also, 'impressed?'

'Did that hurt him? His mouth? It looks a bit cruel,' Melinda asked, with a hint of growing apprehension.

'Only when he tries to run away. Once he stops his behaviour, there is no pressure on his mouth. See, he is just standing here now,' and with that, right on cue, he made another futile attempt to run away. A quick tug on the rope stopped him in his tracks.

'So, Max, if I can get you to hold the lead, and if he tries again, a quick tug will stop him. But not a constant pull. Get it?'

'Sure. I can manage that.'

'While you are holding him, I'll gently inject some

local anaesthetic into the skin around the wound, and then I'll stitch it up, and he will be as good as new.'

I gave the local anaesthetic, which took about 5 minutes to deaden the area. I then quietly stitched the skin edges together. I was indebted to my first and only boss, who had always told me that clients often base their perception of you as a vet on how well you can stitch a wound together. The job took about 15 minutes, and the horse stood still without attempting to run away. Perhaps he realised that his ruse was up, at least with me.

I washed my hands under a nearby tap, collected my instruments, and was good to go.

'Now, Melinda, if you could just keep ...what's your horse's name?'

'Bos.'

'If you could keep him in his paddock for the next two weeks, I'll return to remove the stitches. In the meantime, no riding.'

'I don't ride,' she advised. 'He is actually my brother's horse. He used him for show jumping, but he's having some personal problems and has gone away. So, I'm the bunny. He sometimes sends me money but not for a while...' She didn't finish.

'OK. He's quite a handful for you, with the baby, I mean.'

'Yes,' was her short response, adding, 'in many

ways.'

'So, nobody rides him? That's good in this situation. Exercise would cause the chest muscles to pull on the stitches, and even though I have put two layers in, one underneath and a layer in the skin, they could tear apart if he runs around. OK?'

'I don't think that will be a problem, Rob,' Max said. 'He tends to stand in his shed or his paddock most of the day. He's a bit lazy, and the highlight of his day is when I feed him morning and night.'

'I'll send you a bill, Melinda, unless you want to pay me now,' I said, still feeling uncomfortable about charging.

'An account will help. With the baby and things, my brother's situation. Well, it's tight. But an account will certainly help. I'll pay it as quickly as I can, or when he sends me more money...which may be soon.'

'OK. That's good. When you can...would be much appreciated,' I said as if paying me was, in a way, a gift to me.

On the way back to my car, Max proffered, 'If you don't mind me offering you some advice, young Sir...?'

'Sure. I'd appreciate it, any feedback.'

'I don't know you that well, but I have managed many people in my time, and you are like many employees. The work part comes to you easily; you are good at it, but the money part doesn't. Expect to be paid, Rob, and you will be. And, I have only been in this funny horse agistment business for a short time, but I can tell you that most people I have met actually can't afford horses. But, and this is the important part, they don't know that they can't afford them, and the proverbial hits the fan when there is an unexpected cost.'

'Um...like the vet?' I suggested.

'Yes, like the vet. So, my young friend, if you don't mind me saying, make sure you get paid! At least give them the invoice at the time of service instead of what you offered.'

'I'm a little confused. I did talk about the bill.'

'And gave her...what?' he asked, but I must have looked lost. 'You gave your self a debt, and you gave her credit and almost a license, not to pay you! There wasn't even a time frame for when she thought she could pay. Get it?'

'Putting it that way, I see what you mean. I haven't seen it like that before. Thanks, Max. I'll keep that in mind,' and I sent her an invoice later that day.

As Max had foreseen, when I returned two weeks later to remove the stitches, I had not been paid, and neither had the outstanding agistment bill. Max was right. Eventually, the outstanding account was settled, but not in a way I had foreseen, and Max played a pivotal part.

Rod Graham

Over the next few years, I learned a lot about business from Max.

22 – LIFE'S A LOTTERY

I met Andy one day when I was asked, by a new client to examine, before purchase, a horse that Andy was selling. The sale eventually went through, and in time, Andy became a good mate of mine. He was a top-notch salesman, but like many horse dealers, there was just something that kept him 'on the edge' of true success.

At one point in his illustrious career, so he told me one day, he had worked in a car yard, and a man happened to drive in, asking for directions to the local Mercedes dealership.

The man, Andy realised, wasn't a typical Mercedes' buyer, because, as Andy told me later, 'he didn't look the part.' Andy quickly found out that the man had recently won a lot of money on the lottery, and as Andy related, 'and when I say a lot, I mean, a LOT!' The man left the car yard after buying from Andy, a Range Rover, a double horse float, and a horse, for Andy had discovered what the man had really wanted: a horse! Andy just happened to have one for sale at home. As Andy convinced him, if he had a horse, he would also need a horse float and a Range Rover to pull it.

And that is how I met Bernie, the lottery winner.

Andy introduced me to Bernie and added that I was the 'best horse vet in the world.' Andy sometimes went overboard with his praise, but that was part of what made him a good horse dealer.

Bernie had arrived one day when I was attending Andy's agistment property. He was visiting the new horse that Andy recently sold him. It was one of Andy's retired polo ponies, and instead of just eating its head off for free on Andy's property, it was now still eating its head off, but 'agisted' at Andy's property and paid for by Bernie who didn't ride but just liked horses and had always 'wanted one'.

And Bernie would sit outside the fence, in a rocking chair, and just watch his horse. Sometimes, his wife, Mary, would join him, sit in her chair… and just watch the horse.

And Bernie was happy.

And Andy was happy.

And the horse just kept eating, and so he was happy.

And, each month, Bernie would pay Andy for agisting the horse.

Everyone was happy.

Until one day, the horse stopped eating and stood quietly in the paddock, away from the other horses. And then he started kicking at its stomach and crouching, and jumping forward.

Snippets of a Vet's Life

Bernie was worried. He stopped rocking and stood up.

But Andy wasn't.

'He's just got a bellyache. It will get over it. Give it some sugar cubes.'

Bernie trusted Andy and tried to feed his horse some sugar cubes, but the horse just spat them out. But Andy was wrong. It was more severe than a bellyache. The horse started to lie down and attempt to roll over.

'Don't let him do that!' Andy volunteered. 'He could twist his gut.'

'How do we stop him from rolling?' Bernie asked, somewhat alarmed.

'Walk him, and when he tries to get down, make a noise and move him on; otherwise, he may die.'

Bernie and his wife were now very alarmed.

They had grown close to their horse and didn't want him to suffer. Being new horse owners, they relied a lot on Andy and followed whatever Andy advised them to do. But Andy was not a vet.

'You'd better call in Rob, because he's the best vet in the world, and if anybody can save your horse, Rob can.'

He then told them that he had to leave, jumped in his car, and drove out the gate, yelling, 'Don't let the horse roll!'

Rod Graham

Driving to Andy's agistment property on the other side of the city took about an hour, and by the time I arrived, Bernie was quite upset and distressed. Despite their best efforts, he and his wife were not always able to prevent their horse from violently throwing itself on the ground and rolling over. To make matters worse, the horse had got itself caught under a fence and had injured its front leg.

As I got out of my car, Bernie ran over. 'Thank you for coming. We are very worried. Will he be alright?' I immediately liked him because he used the magic words, 'Thank you.' Not always used, but a simple acknowledgement of one person's effort by another never goes astray.

I listened to the horse's heart rate. It was high. I listen to the horse's gut sound with my stethoscope. First on the left side, then on the right side of the abdomen. A 'tinkle, tinkle' sound was all I could hear.

I checked the horse's gum colour. It was very red, and when I put pressure on the gum with my finger, the blood quickly returned after I removed my finger. Being a horse vet is somewhat akin to being an involuntary thrill-seeker at times, and this was one of those moments. I now needed to examine the horse internally by putting my lubricated right arm through the horse's rectum and using the lower bowel as a sleeve to feel what was happening inside the horse's abdomen.

Snippets of a Vet's Life

Unless the horse was restrained, there was a good chance that I could be kicked.

'OK,' I said. 'What I want you to do, Bernie, is I want you to hold the horse's head so he can't go forward, and Mary, I want you to push against his hip and flanks against the wall so he can't move sideways while I try to examine him internally.' Surprisingly, they did as I had instructed, and this allowed me to do an internal examination without getting kicked by the horse.

What I felt was not encouraging. I couldn't get very far into the abdomen because loops of gas-filled intestines hindered my exploring arm's progress. I removed my arm and took off the examination glove.

'I have to do one further test.'

Once again, I got Bernie and Mary into their previous positions, again retraining the horse against a wall. This time, I took a 10cm 18g stainless steel hypodermic needle and positioned it underneath the horse's abdomen, near the belly button. With a quick tap, I punched the tip through the wall of the abdomen so that now the tip was inside the wall of the abdomen, and the other end was outside the skin.

I didn't have long to wait until I saw what I had feared. Yellow abdominal fluid tinged with blood drained out of the external end of the needle. And not just a few drops, but a lot freely flowed. A 'lot' usually meant that a damaged part of the intestines was leaking fluid.

'This is not good. I am fairly certain that your horse has a twisted gut. And for him to have any chance, he will need surgery.'

'Can you do that? Can you fix him?' Bernie asked.

'No, I can't. Not in the paddock. We need to get him to the University if he's to have a chance, but even then, his chance of surviving is slim.'

As a student, I had assisted with many late-night colic surgeries at the University, and I knew that what increased the chances of success was the speed with which the open abdomen surgery occurred and the damage to the intestines was rectified.

'I will give him a powerful painkiller, and he will seem better, but that is just because I am covering up the pain for the trip. Let's get him on the float and get you on your way.'

'What about the cut on his leg?'.

'They will fix that during the colic surgery.'

'Is he going to die?'

'I don't know, but you need to get going quickly now.'

This was a time before Google Maps. I drew them simple directions on a piece of paper. Before the 'big win' changed his life, Bernie had been a truck driver, and he knew where to go.

Snippets of a Vet's Life

Bernie's horse didn't die, and about two weeks later, the horse was discharged from the university and brought back to Andy's agistment property.

Regularly deworming a horse is strongly linked to reducing the risk of colic. I explained this to Bernie and arranged to meet him the following weekend at Andy's property.

'There will be two horses for you to worm, Rob,' announced Bernie. 'Andy told me that he thought that my horse got colic because he was missing his brother, and Andy had found his brother by chance the other day, so I bought him.'

'So, you now have two? And did Andy say where he found his brother?'

'Well. This is the amazing part. Andy happened to be at the horse sales last week, and the horse came into the sale ring, so Andy bought him for me.'

'How did Andy know that they were brothers?'.

'Don't know. But Andy just knows these things. Just like he knew you were a good vet.'

'See you Saturday?'

'Yep.'

'And Rob...Thanks.'

Saying that is always welcomed by a vet.

23 – A COW SUDDENLY DIES

Let's be honest: I was not very experienced in the Sudden Death of Cattle syndrome, or for that matter, cows in any state of health.

I straightened up after examining the dead animal.

'It may be 'bloat' or perhaps snakebite, and because there was a thunderstorm yesterday, perhaps lightning strike, or...' and I paused, searching my memory for the other causes of sudden death in cattle.

One of the skills that a vet gradually learns is to be an observer of the little things when analysing a situation.

'But a lightning strike is unlikely because I can't see any burn marks on its coat. ' I paused, 'There can be other causes...'

And it was one of the other causes that had me worried.

I wondered if it was possibly Anthrax, a disease caused by Bacillus bacteria that can infect and kill humans and other animals. I surmised that even though the syndrome is called 'Sudden Death', the death is rarely sudden. What is often observed is that a cow is grazing peacefully in a paddock one day and is found dead the After examining the luckless beast, I decided to dive straight in.

'Since the diagnosis is a bit open, and there are other cattle I see in the same field, I'd like to send a sample off to the Government Laboratory to check if that is OK with you, Mrs Pridham? All I need to do is cut off an ear and send it to the lab,' without adding that this was what I remembered from a long-ago lecture.

Len, her farm manager, sceptically asked, 'Do you think that is really necessary? Look at her abdomen; it looks to me like bloat.' It was true, the dead cow's abdomen was enlarged.

'I see what you mean, but gases build up after death, no matter what the cause, so I don't think we can make a diagnosis of bloat. To be honest, Mrs Pridham, Len, I don't treat a lot of cows, mostly horses, and so I am a bit out of my depth when it comes to cow diseases.'

'Len. If he thinks we should do it, then let us do it,' She spoke with quiet authority, and in response, Len indicated his acquiescence by gently bowing his head in her direction. And I was her tenant… for effectively nothing. So when Len contacted me that morning for help, I agreed to help. And as I considered how much harm could I cause by looking at her dead cow?

'It's good of you to help us, Dr. McBride. We normally use Dr. Aiken for our cattle work, but I'm not sure if you know that he is not currently available. So, any insight you have would be most appreciated,' said Mrs Pridham.

I secretly remembered how my earlier rabies diagnosis, when I was a very new veterinarian, had alarmed an elderly lady. The alarming diagnosis had also come out of my need to 'not miss something really serious', which is a common fear of young vets.

I did not want to alarm another older lady who was standing in front of me, and who just happened to be my landlady.

The good lady and I had an interesting but always formal relationship. I only saw the person behind the reserve once.

I had been invited to Christmas Drinks at her home, Emmerton House. Whilst she and I were standing on the back balcony that overlooked the vegetable garden and green fields beyond, she said, for no apparent reason, 'Do you realise, Rob, that I have lived in other people's mansions all my life, and now I have a home?' I turned and looked at her. But she kept her gaze steady and looked into the far distance. Just silence, and then abruptly she turned and walked inside, back to her waiting guests.

My thoughts returned to the task at hand. I put on sterile gloves and, with a scalpel, I severed the ear from the hapless dead cow, and as I did so, the summer flies swarmed on the dark red oozing blood.

Snippets of a Vet's Life

If a vet suspected they were dealing with a potential case of Anthrax, there was an Agricultural Department protocol to follow. It started with severing the ear of the dead animal. I put the ear in a plastic bag, sealed it as best I could, and later, after placing the plastic bag and ear in a watertight large envelope, I gave my package to the train guard at Coldstream Station and dispatched the severed ear to the Veterinary Research Institute in Parkville, Melbourne.

I knew that the blood oozing from the severed ear would be examined under a microscope, and the laboratory scientist would look for telltale signs of the deadly bacteria.

As part of the admissions protocol, I completed a form with the required information, including the property's history, location, and owner. In the case notes section, I wrote the brief words, 'Right ear from a 4-year-old cow. Sudden Death,' and added, almost as an afterthought, 'Is it Anthrax?'

Not much happened at work the following day, so I went swimming. On returning, I felt very relaxed and refreshed, and I casually wandered up the steps and into my office.

'Hi,' I said to Joan as I entered the door.

'You're finally back!' she exclaimed before I could ask her anything. She had a flustered look on her face.

'There is an urgent phone call. From the head of the Agricultural Department. Something about a cow.... a dead cow?'

My relaxed feeling left and was replaced with alarm.

So I was right! It was anthrax, or so I thought, as I quickly dialled the number and asked for the Chief Veterinary Officer of Victoria.

A woman answered, and I was put on hold after explaining who I was. Whilst waiting for the Chief Vet to answer, I wondered *why would the Head Government Vet want to talk to me*? I assumed that it had something to do with my Anthrax query. But why was I speaking with such a highly placed government official? Couldn't a laboratory technician give me the report? Or a laboratory vet?

'Is that you, Rob?' asked an older sounding man, gruffly.

'Hello. Yes, I'm Rob..... how can I help you?'

'About that submission, the suspect anthrax case that you sent yesterday to the Government Laboratory, on the train, with no warning, and not suitably packaged for transport.'

'Yes...?' I responded cautiously and then quickly thought, 'Oops.'

This conversation was turning a bit 'nasty', and it had only just started.

'Do you do much cattle work, Rob?' he asked.

'Ah ... no. I'm a horse vet.'

Snippets of a Vet's Life

'Then that explains it, Rob,' and before I could go on to ask, 'explains, what?' he asked another question.

'Do you know what happens to an area if we have, or are suspicious of, or if...' he paused and then continued, accentuating his words, 'a *competent* vet is suspicious of an outbreak of anthrax?'

I was beginning to understand where this conversation was going.

'No, I don't, actually,' and I was starting to feel angry at his manner.

'Well, I will tell you. We physically close the area down, Rob. And in this case, it would mean the Yarra Valley. There would be roadblocks. Nobody allowed in or out, without first going through a cleansing process, and no movement of any ANIMALS,' and he paused to give gravity to what he was saying.

'That's what we do if there is a suspicion of Anthrax. So, Rob, before I implement that protocol and order the Yarra Valley to be isolated, and because the outbreak is so close to metropolitan Melbourne, alert the Police, and while we are waiting on the result from the lab, do you have a serious concern that you are dealing with anthrax?'

But that wasn't the end of it. Secretly, I marvelled at his ability, with words, to succinctly put the case to me.

'Well. Um. Not sure. As I said, I usually just see horses, and my landlady had a dead cow, and I thought

I was doing the right thing. Perhaps it was 'bloat' after all. I just didn't want to miss Anthrax.'

Bloat is a condition in cattle in which the main, large stomach, called the rumen, expands because of the buildup of digestive gases. It can happen at any time in life for various reasons, but it always happens after a cow dies.

'You mentioned your landlady. Is that the person nominated on the admission form as the owner of the farm under suspicion?'

'Yes. Pamela Pridham,' I replied.

'And do you know if she is connected to the same family who runs Wave Hill Station in the Northern Territory?' he paused, took a breath and added,' and other beef-producing properties in the North?'

I mumbled an affirmative, and I was beginning to see that there was now a political element to our conversation and why the Chief Government Vet was talking to me. At this stage, a pastoral company, based in the UK and controlled by Mrs Pridham's family, owned the lease for a large swathe of the Northern Territory, including Wave Hill Station, the site of the now famous 'Walk Off' by the First Nation workers.

On 23 August 1966, 200 Gurindji stock-men and Wave Hill employees withheld their labour to demand better pay and working conditions. Their action is considered the start of the 'Aboriginal Rights' movement, culminating in the now famous 'Land

Rights' Mabo Case in the High Court, handed down in 1992, granting Native Title over certain lands.

So, after the Wave Hill walk-off, any connection to the family involved was on the 'Public Radar.'

What would have happened if the Melbourne media had got wind of what I potentially had diagnosed? I envisaged 'Anthrax Hits Largest Beef Exporter in Australia!' would possibly be that evening's Headline News.

Due to the family connection, if the information that there was an outbreak of anthrax on one of their properties had been leaked to the news media, it could have significantly impacted the export livestock market and potentially caused the Australian economy to lose millions of dollars in exports.

Was this why the Chief Veterinary Officer was handling this matter?

'One final thing, Rob'

'Yes?'

'If I were you, I would stay a horse vet and leave the cow work to somebody who knows what they are doing!'

I thanked him for his advice, even though I thought he was a bit unfair. But I got the message: stick to what I know. But what if it had been Anthrax?

The following day, I received the result: 'negative' for anthrax.

Rod Graham

After getting the negative feedback, I rarely examined cows again, and as a result, the Australian economy continued without my intervention.

But, one way or another, cows have been an issue for me.

24 – ORAL EXAMS, IN PARTICULAR: COWS

During my first year, my dislike of treating cows gradually grew, as my fondness for horses was reinforced, which was the primary reason that later, I became a horse vet.

Years earlier, I had chosen to attend my school because it was agriculturally focused, and I had developed a wish to be a dairy farmer.

During school holidays, and as was expected, I spent a summer working on a dairy farm. Didn't I want to be a dairy farmer? But I concluded that I did not have what it took to be a dairy farmer, even though that had been why I had chosen to go to this school.

Between the early start to milk them, the relentless need to milk them twice a day, their ability to spray urine and faeces on you, even from a distance, and their ability to hit you across your face with their wet urine-laden tail and their attraction to flies, and in particular blow flies, all this, put together, I think this is why I fell out of love with cows that summer.

Luckily, I became distracted by a desire to be a veterinarian, but I was not done with cow contact. There were many lectures on cows and their diseases.

It was final exam time at Veterinary school, and part of the process involved oral examinations with various department heads. I had fared well, or so I thought, which was a warning.

Why? If a student felt that they had done well, there were two possibilities:

1. You actually knew a lot and were probably a nerd

2. You did not know how much you didn't know and hence did not realise that your answers were a 'bit light on'.

I was worried, who was I? Nerd, or dumb?

The last oral worried me in particular, and it was with Professor Blood, who also happened to be the Head of the Bovine (cow) division. Coincidentally, the administrative Head of School at this stage was Colin Bone, so we always said that Blood and Bone ran the Vet School.

Bovine medicine awaited: At the very least, a pass was needed for me to graduate and be registered as a vet.

I knocked on the Professor's door. My hands were clammy, and my heart rate was up. I was very nervous.

'Come in,' came from behind the door.

Snippets of a Vet's Life

I walked in and sat down in front of the Professor. Behind him was a painting of cows. I suspected that the Professor liked cows. I didn't dislike cows, but I didn't see my veterinary career heading in that direction. I was a lacking a bit in knowledge when it came to the diseases and ailments of cows.

'So, Rob, let's start by you telling me all you know about mastitis.'

I felt inwardly smug. I had predicted this question and knew it well. I rattled off my knowledge, gained the night before in preparation, of mastitis, which is the inflammation of the cow's udder. But before I could comfortably continue with that answer, I was interrupted by a new question.

'OK, Rob. Very good. You seem to know that. But what can you tell me...?' and he nominated the next topic and then the next.

I blundered through as best I could and felt that I was just keeping my head above water, but I now realise that he was more interested in how much I did NOT know. His questions revealed serious gaps in my knowledge of the disease and ailments of cows.

'OK, Rob,' he said, looking at the clock, 'we are coming to the end, and I just have one last question. ' He had my complete attention.

'Tell me what you know about white muscle disease in calves?'

'Well. White muscle disease,' and I paused, playing for time, 'A key element of the white muscle disease is a lack of vitamin E and ...' (To be truthful, I should have answered, 'Not a lot' to his question, 'tell me what you know'.)

'Are you thinking of Selenium, Rob? Go on...'

'Yes. Thank you. Yes, selenium.' I started padding. 'And one area noted for this disease is the Coorong area of South Australia.'

'Why?' he shot back.

'Because the soils are deficient in selenium?

'Very good, Rob, but I am more interested in how the two forms of the disease present.'

That was news to me: two forms. I was about to answer with some made up gibberish, basically still playing for time, when we both heard frantic knocking on the door.

'Yes?' the Professor said sharply, perhaps somewhat irritated at my lack of knowledge, or that we were being interrupted.

His secretary barged into the room with a startled look on her face.

'He's been sacked!' she excitedly announced. 'The Governor General has acted and sacked Whitlam.'

We both looked at her, processing what she had just reported, and then the Professor looked back at me and said, 'OK. Rob. I think we will end it there.' He stood up and quickly left the room.

As the history books now record, in the early afternoon of 11 November 1975, and after a series of dramatic events, including a 1974 double dissolution and a budgetary supply crisis, the Gough Whitlam led federal Labor government became the first (and only) government in Australian history to be dismissed by the Governor General.

His actions also had a lasting effect on my veterinary career.

The Governor General's dramatic decision had not 'curdled my milk'. And as I later learned, I had just 'skimmed' through bovine medicine with a bare 'pass'.

But it was enough for me to qualify as a veterinarian.

25 – THE FAVOURITE

He had the body of a Percheron crossed with that of a thoroughbred, but he had the mind of a Shetland pony.

'Bos' was his name.

He became mine as payment for a debt. As described I had been called to Max McClintock's agistment property, Happy Acres, a few weeks earlier to stitch a horse that had cut its chest. After completing the task, I provided his owner with an account. As Max had prophesied, I had created a problem for myself: how NOT to get paid.

Later, with Max's intercession, I made a deal with the owner's sister, whom I had met a few weeks earlier. After forgoing the debt owed to me and parting with money, most of which was used to discharge the unpaid agistment debt owed to Max's wife Anne, I became the new owner of Bos.

One specific issue I inherited from his previous owner was Bos's reluctance to travel in a horse float or trailer. On one occasion, apparently, his last owner, the brother, had used some force to coerce him into the float by employing a stock whip. Once they started their journey, Bos destroyed the float by relentlessly kicking at the sides and the back ramp. He was also hard to lead along a lane-way, often flipping his head and running away.

As a result, Bos had a bad reputation, which probably explained Max's comment that I would have a few problems getting him onto a float.

'As you know, my young friend, he has 'attitude', Max volunteered while I was preparing to transport him, after the sale, from Happy Acres to the Green Cottage.

When I attempted to load him onto a horse float for the first time, and as he stepped on the tail ramp, he quickly turned his head the other way, using the strength of his neck, pulled the lead out of my hands, and attempted to run away. But Max, ever the pessimist, always held the belief that if things could go wrong with horses and their owners, they would. Fortunately, he had closed the lane-way gate, and Bos could not run far. I retrieved him.

This was his 'thing': his strategy of avoiding whatever he did not want to do at the time. And it was apparent he did not want to get into the horse float, or for that matter, even approach it. A quick sideways shift of his head and then running away had always worked for him, so he continued to use it. He did not realise that, as a result, more stringent measures were often employed to get him onto a float/horsebox.

Managing horses is often like managing children: given some thought, you can often out think them.

Bos stood like a statue, but the flick of his ear and a slight shifting of his weight told me that he was worried. Before the next attempt to walk him towards the float, I threaded the lead from the clip through the other side of his mouth and back into my hands. I as when I first met him a few weeks earlier. We approached the loading ramp, and Bos did his usual trick of throwing his head away from me. This time, I was ready and had looped the rope lead through his mouth. His attempt to pull the rope out of my hands caused him some discomfort in his mouth, and I could pull his head back around to face the float, thus stopping him from running away.

'Well. That seems to be a wake-up for him, Rob.' Max said with a 'let's see how successful you are at getting actually on the float' look on his face.

With me leading, Bos and I approached the loading ramp again. At the same time, I was jiggling the lead, letting him know that I was in control of his mouth. He put his front feet on the ramp and came to a stop. Clearly, he thought about running away, but he couldn't since I had control of his mouth. He stood there, and I stood alongside him. We both waited. He looked at me. I looked back.

Snippets of a Vet's Life

Impasse?

I patiently waited.

Finally, he took a big breath and, on exhaling, walked into the float.

From then on, I found that if I gave him time to think about getting into the float, there was usually no problem, but if I tried to hurry him on, he resisted. In this way, he was very human: acknowledging and expressing free will. I understood this need and gave him time to consider. This is why we bonded. I understood him.

He was at times clever, slightly devious, and mischievous, just like a naughty Shetland pony.

But he was, by nature, lazy. If given the choice of looking sleek, fit, vibrant and bold, or fat and sedentary with the merest flicker of his ears at the annoying flies being the total of the day's exercise, Bos would always choose the latter.

Once a year, usually in autumn, when I started getting him fit for winter, we would jog in one direction. Then, ever so swiftly, he'd go in the opposite direction, back towards his paddock, almost with a look of glee on his face, leaving me on the ground, struggling to get up, facing a long walk home.

In time, he seemingly realised that the jingle of the stirrups, as I carried the saddle out the back door, in association with the distinctive sound of closing the back door, heralded my arrival in his paddock to catch him for a ride.

In response to these sounds, he would stop whatever he was doing, which often was grazing, walk towards the only tree growing in the centre of his five acre paddock, and then stand with his head on the other side of the thick tree trunk. He probably thought I could not see him if he could not see me. How else could I explain this routine behaviour?

In many ways, he was clever, but not that clever. His head may have been hidden, but the rest of his body was evident as I opened the gate into his paddock. Putting the saddle down, I would quietly walk towards him and then jump from around the tree trunk in front of him. He always got a fright, and I am sure he never worked out how I discovered him each time.

In a way, he acted at times like a naughty little boy.

One night, I was soundly asleep when I heard a strange noise outside my bedroom window. It sounded as though I had an unwelcome guest walking on the verandah. I dressed, thinking it was an intruder, and did not turn on any lights. I quietly exited the back door, trying not to make a sound. I crept around the corner and shone a light where I had judged the intruder to be. No intruder in the torchlight but the large eyes of a chestnut horse's head. It was Bos on the verandah. And I assumed he had been walking along the verandah to get to the bag of horse feed outside the dining room window. He got a fright from the torch, startled, and turned about face, running back the way he had come and then back towards his paddock. I was lucky that his weight had not broken through the verandah floorboards. He could have easily damaged himself had he caught his leg.

It was a warning always to make sure his gate was closed.

The following day, I attached a self-closing mechanism to his gate, and from then on, Bos did not attempt to visit the horse larder late at night.

Later in life, he developed an arthritic condition in his front legs, known as 'ringbone'. Initially, he was only slightly lame, but as the bony changes destroyed more of the shiny part of his pastern joints, the lameness became more permanent, and I retired him from active use.

He lived out his life on Joan's farm until one day she contacted me to let me know she had 'made the hard decision and had him put down.'

She had not contacted me before this happened because she was trying to spare me the 'pain' of the decision. I was genuinely shocked.

I didn't have the opportunity to say goodbye, but I was also aware that Joan, who ran the office, was genuinely thinking of me. I thanked her for what she had done and grieved quietly, away from her.

My own experience of this ongoing 'loss' has guided my advice to owners making similar decisions at the end of a much-loved pet's life. Include every family member in the decision-making process, even if they are overseas or interstate.

Sometimes, adult children, who are far away, may want a keepsake of an old dog or cat that was a childhood pet, if given notice. You just can't predict how others will react.

Include them.

I have owned many horses over the years, but Bos has remained my favourite, and I still remember him many years after his death.

And I still miss him…and his naughty ways.

26 – ENTER COLUMBINA, STAGE LEFT

I remember the day I first met Victoria and Tim as clearly as I remember my first solo stitching of a horse's wound. I met them in late spring, on the sort of afternoon where the sun hovers and everything smells like freshly mowed pastures and newly born lambs.

On returning from breakfast at the local petrol station, the answering machine was blinking, indicating a recent contact. I returned the call.

A woman's voice, crisp and unhurried, answered. 'Broomhill. Hello?' 'Hi. You left a message for me? I'm Dr Rob.'

'Is this the young vet?'

'Yes, this is Rob.'

'We've had a situation. An unexpected delivery.'

'Delivery of what?'

'A baby donkey. Our Columbina has just given birth overnight. I think the placenta's retained. We could use your help.'

She gave the address, then added, almost as an

afterthought, 'Forgive my rudeness for not introducing myself. I'm Victoria. And you will meet my husband, Tim. He's calm in emergencies but has a tendency to quote Shakespeare under pressure. Don't be alarmed.'

'That's OK, because I tend to quote The Great Gatsby,' I said, perhaps a bit light-heartedly.

'Oh' was all she said.

I drove up the winding gravel road to Broomhill Farm, feeling more nervous than usual about meeting new clients. I'd dealt with horses, goats, and even an emu once. But donkeys? Not many, except the occasional one standing in a swimming pool. Many people think of donkeys as slightly different horses. But they are not. They have a very different mindset. A horse will often be forgiving, or possibly, forgetful. Donkeys always remember and sometimes hold grudges, and they kick without warning.

The paddock was a picture. Rolling grass, an old stable leaning slightly to one side, and in the middle, a donkey foal lying in a patch of hay. Her mother, large, light grey, and not remotely bothered by my arrival, stood nearby, munching steadily.

Victoria met me at the gate. Linen smock, and smudges of charcoal on her hands. Was she an artist? I wondered. She had the worried look of someone who'd already imagined five different outcomes.

'How long ago was the birth?'

Snippets of a Vet's Life

'Last night she foaled. All was quiet until we noticed the afterbirth hadn't passed.'

'And this is her first foal?'

'As far as we know. She escaped a few months ago, and we now know why.'

'So that's when you think she got pregnant?'

'Must have been. Tim is calling the foal Tulip, because she arrived like a bloom.'

'Clever.'

A man, whom I assumed was Tim, appeared then, trailing hay and without an apparent need, proclaimed, with a dramatic flair, 'A miracle among mortals, and yet, nature trembles.'

'Hi. I'm Rob. Was that Shakespeare?' I asked, remembering how his wife had described her husband.

'No. Me! Greetings to you, young vet!' he said, beaming, and extending his hand in welcome. 'Victoria said you'd have excellent hair and an earnest gait.'

I wondered about his statement. Sounded a bit weird, since Victoria and I had only just met.

I turned my attention to the patient Columbina. Her flanks twitched. Her eyes were calm but alert. I gave her a gentle examination and confirmed what Victoria suspected. The placenta was retained: it was still inside her womb.

'We'll need to help her pass it. Some oxytocin should

do the trick. Might need antibiotics after, just in case.'

'Do what you need,' Victoria said. 'She is like a family member. You'll be gentle?'

I nodded.

'Always.'

The procedure was straightforward enough. I washed and sterilised my hands and arms, and pulled gently on part of the retained afterbirth that was hanging from her birth passage. Columbina tolerated me, any intrusion. With a constant pull, the placenta passed, and I felt a wave of relief.

'That's it. She should be fine now.'

'Thank you,' Victoria said softly.

'Will she bond with the foal?' Tim asked.

'Looks like she already has. She's attentive. The foal is nursing well. That's all we want for now.'

Victoria walked me back to the gate.

'Columbina came with no name when she was only 6 weeks old. She was a wedding anniversary present from Tim, years ago. Can't remember how many, but it was well before we retired,' she said, glancing back at the donkey. 'But I've been thinking... Columbina. Tim named her. You understand the name? Like the Commedia dell'arte character. Always watchful. And witty. Sometimes devious, and always desirable, plus full of unspoken wisdom.'

Snippets of a Vet's Life

'Oh.' I was at a loss, unsure what a Commedia dell'arte character was. So I just replied with, 'It suits her.'

'I think so too. She has wisdom '

'And Tulip?'

'An accident. But a beautiful one.'

We stood for a moment, watching the mother and foal. 'Thank you for calling me. It has been a pleasure meeting you both...and Columbina,' I said.

'You came when we called, and that's what matters.'

Victoria hesitated as I reached for the car door.

'Would you like a cup of tea or coffee, and I have just baked some lamingtons.'

It was the mention of lamingtons, my favourite cake, and the openness of these two people that enticed me to consider how to answer. I paused. My instinct was to politely decline. Keep it professional. On to the next call. But there was something in her tone, open, warm, almost hopeful.

I mused and realised that, paraphrasing a line from The Great Gatsby, they had a simplicity of heart that was its own ticket of admission.

'I'd like that,' I said.

The kitchen was full of light. Big windows, terracotta tiles, wooden benches worn smooth with age. It smelled like rosemary and charcoal pencils.

Tim poured the coffee, humming something from a musical I half recognised. Victoria handed me a plate of lamingtons.

'Great. My favourite. I haven't had lamingtons for a long time...last time I was home.'

'It's nice to sit after everything,' she said. 'Columbina. She's a magnificent creature, isn't she? I think she knew you meant well.'

'You think so? Perhaps. Maybe.'

'No, I'm sure. Columbina is wise. I know.'

I sat at the long pine table; hands wrapped around the warm mug. They asked about how long I'd been there and if I needed some help. I told them how my funny little practice had started after leaving my job with Doug. I admitted I was mostly alone. Just me and Joan, who worked part-time, and that we ran the practice out of the Green Cottage.

'Girlfriend?'

'No. I'm not very good when it comes to girls.'

'That must get lonely,' Victoria said gently.

I hesitated. Most people didn't notice. Or if they did, they didn't say it out loud.

'It does, sometimes.'

Tim nodded.

'We know a little about that. Retiring is a strange thing. Your calendar empties, but your thoughts don't.

Snippets of a Vet's Life

I was the school head of drama, but they got rid of me.' There was a hint of resentment in his voice.

'And friends your own age don't always want to talk about donkeys and duck digestion,' Victoria added with a smile.

I laughed.

'Exactly.'

We chatted for over an hour about art, theatre, animals, weather, books, and ridiculous situations that a young vet finds themselves in. I briefly mentioned my student days and my childhood. Private stuff that I normally kept to myself. It was easier than I'd expected. They weren't trying to parent or impress me. They just... welcomed me.

When I finally stood to go, Victoria offered me a small jar of homemade plum jam.

'Take this. And come back, even if there's no emergency.'

And through the open window, I heard Columbina bray.

Just once. Low and satisfied, the sound perhaps of a new mother.

'I think she approves, 'Victoria said and as I stood to leave. She handed me my vet bag.

'Thanks. I doubt that she would give me a second thought.'

As I walked back to the car, I felt a quiet calm. Not because of the successful procedure, or the lamingtons, though both helped, but because I genuinely like these older people.

As I reached the car, Tim called after me.

'You will come back, won't you? We have a cockatoo with emotional issues, hens with theatrical leanings, and ducks who always argue. And a wife who has an opinion on all of it, and me, a retired thespian. Perhaps one night for dinner?'

'Sounds like I don't have a choice. But Tim, I mostly work with horses... and donkeys. Not sure I would be much use with cockatoos, hens and ducks, but I'm always happy to help if I can.'

'Indeed! All the world's a stage, and yours is Broomhill,' Tim replied as if this were an everyday observation.

I laughed.

That night, I pulled off my boots and dropped onto the couch. Then I noticed something.

My vet bag lay open in the hallway, where I had unconsciously dropped it. Something white caught my attention.

Inside, on top of the stethoscope and thermometer, was a small white towel and three lamingtons.

I looked out the window, toward the rising moon, and wondered: What did I know now about goats or ducks?

Snippets of a Vet's Life

And who were these people, the artist and the drama teacher?

And Columbina, a donkey whose patient gaze seemed to dare me to see more than I was seeing.

27 – THE MOTHER OF ALL HOLIDAYS

In time, word of me spread. Under Joan's financial guidance and my hard work, the practice grew. And in time, and to make my life more manageable, I employed Vicky as a part-time housekeeper plus office assistant to Joan.

Vicky was originally a client and had sought my help for a lame horse.

I met her in the most unusual circumstances, while underneath the Green Cottage. One Saturday afternoon, I was using a car jack to lift the cottage frame onto bricks so that I could open the cottage front door.

I was well and truly wedged under the cottage when I heard the front gate make its characteristic scraping noise. Then silence. I listened. Nothing. Then I heard somebody cautiously walking above on the verandah floorboards-step by hesitant step.

'Hello,' I yelled out.

'I'm looking for Rob...the vet' was the muffled reply from a female voice that I did not recognise.

'That's me. What do you want?'

Snippets of a Vet's Life

I couldn't quite hear her answer clearly, so I yelled out, 'Come around to the other side of the house. I'm underneath.'

You are probably wondering why I did not remove myself from under the Cottage, do the right thing, and greet my visitor as any normal person would. I'm wondering that now myself, but I didn't. I do remember that there was not a lot of space under the floorboards at the front of the cottage, and it had taken me some effort to crawl there.

Perhaps that is why I said, 'Look, I'm under the house, and it is a bit hard to crawl out unless it is important. Do you have a sick horse?'

'No. He's lame. Don't crawl out,' my visitor yelled back. 'It is not that important.'

'Sure?

'I can wait.'

'If you want, why don't you crawl under the house a bit so that we can talk?'

Even I can now recognise that there was something slightly *wicked* about me at this stage of my life.

And that is how I met Vicky. I'm not one for clothes usually, but I did notice that she wore a white pantsuit at the time. Vicky proved to be a God-send, and apart from housekeeping the Green Cottage, at the office, she would answer the phone, make bookings, help Joan, and with some training, Vicky I discovered, had a hidden ability to differentiate the various type of blood cells viewed under a microscope. And with a bit of training she was able to help process the many blood tests required by our horse trainer clients.

Vicky also helped take care of my horse, and it was because he was injured that I received a call early one morning, while asleep in London.

I was finally able to go overseas for the holiday that Joan had often talked about, and though I had increasingly needed to take.

I had given up attempting to have a holiday locally. I just could not get away from the need to be in contact. Then, all that changed when, acting on Joan's advice, I bought a ticket and, with no plans, headed for the UK and Ireland. As I settled into the cattle-class seat of the aeroplane, for the first time in a long while, I felt comfortable about taking a holiday.

A lot happened on that holiday and I was truly relaxed and enjoying my time, even though it was costing me a lot of money.

About a week into in my planned four week stay, I received the phone call from reception in the early morning while staying at a cheap hotel in London.

'Yes?'

'Mr McBride. We have a call from Melbourne, Australia. Will you accept it?'

Realising that there was no other answer, I replied,

Snippets of a Vet's Life

'Yes.'

From the phone came this question, 'Is that you?' I recognised her voice.

'Vicky. How are you? How did you find me?'

I felt intruded upon, and perhaps sounded a bit angry and put out. Before I got married and took on family responsibilities, I was somewhat vague about where I would be during my holidays. At that stage of my life, I was quite paranoid about privacy.

'How did you find me?' I repeated tersely. I was amazed at how she managed to locate me on the other side of the world, in a hotel room in London, with so few clues. I never did find out how she located me. But she did because my horse, Bos, was injured in a storm, and Vicky wanted to know which vet I would prefer.

'Get Gerald. Thanks.' Gerald was a trusted colleague of mine and a highly skilled horse veterinarian.

Click, and I went back to sleep.

The following day, I was out riding in Leicestershire, north of London, and at times mixing with people who never seemed to have to work. But this idyllic sojourn was not to last.

About two weeks later, a late-night phone call, this time from Joan, brought me back to reality and to work. A small problem with the bank was how she described it, and I just knew she would be moving her mouth in that tight side-to-side way she did whenever she was stressed.

'Can you say more?'

'Not over the phone, dear.'

So, I returned, and the following morning, still a bit jet-lagged, I greeted Joan and then asked why she had called me back.

'You said that there was a small problem with the back? What's wrong?'

There seemed to be a lot of money in my account, which was lucky because where I was staying, and the people I was meeting, well… let's just say, they lived life at a level beyond my pay grade.

'That's good, dear. As they came in, I continued to deposit the cheques into your private account. I thought you might need the extra money.'

I thought about this for a moment.

'So… what's the state of the practice account?' I asked, maybe a little worried.

'Slight problem there. Funds are a bit low. I haven't been able to pay creditors for a week. But… once I told them that you're overseas and will fix it all when you get back, most of them have been okay, except the petrol man, Ken. He wants cash before he will fill up your car. And, there is one other thing. The overdraft has blown out, and that's probably why the cheque I gave to the petrol man bounced recently. The bank manager wants you to give him a call this morning.'

'He does?' I felt a bit overwhelmed, as if I'd been hit by a ten-ton truck.

'Yes, as soon as possible, were his exact words.'

'Oh.' I felt sick.

'Welcome back, Boss!' and she put her head down, and went about her work.

Rod Graham

28 – WAGER: WHO LET THE HOUND IN?

It started with a question.

'Would you like to give a retired foxhound a home?'

Max McClintock gave one of those slow nods, the kind that offered no real answer, but then again, it wasn't a 'no'.

'Maybe. We'll see.'

And that was it. It was enough.

Two days later, I arrived with Wager.

He had been part of a local pack of foxhounds, but he was getting old. A younger hound had turned on him, grabbed him by the back of his neck, and had the hound man not acted quickly, Wager would have been killed by the pack. Such is the fate of old animals that live in a pack.

'Can't have that, Rob. Can't have them fighting. May have to put him down,' was Tom's pronouncement. Tom was a man of few words, but we seemed to get along OK. He had called me out to tend to his horse, and then asked, as I was about to leave, 'While you are here,

Snippets of a Vet's Life

Rob, can you look at Wager?

'Give me a day or two, and I'll see if I can find him a home. Shouldn't be too hard around here.'

'OK. But don't take too long, if you get my drift.'

Wager was rangy and strong, with ears like battered leather. His black and tan coat had scars from past encounters, but he was still agile, ever alert and ready to join the pack. In truth, he'd been retired for a reason. Too headstrong, they said, as he got older. Didn't work well in the pack. His days seemed to be numbered. As I patted him, he responded. I liked him. I thought he'd do well in a quieter place.

I thought of Max and Anne. To this day, I'm not sure why, probably because Wager, the fox hound reminded me of Max, the man.

They had the land and the space. And they did not have a dog. They had a cat, but Max rarely saw it, and it tended to live in the stables. When I offered, Anne had seemed mildly interested. Max just said, 'We'll see.'

But when I turned up with Wager sitting upright in the backseat of my car, they didn't turn me away.

That had been a few weeks earlier, and this day I was calling in to check on a lame pony at a neighbouring property, and I thought I'd drop by.

Anne answered the door. She was wearing her gardening gloves and holding a broken flowerpot.

'Hello, Robert...that Wager! He's chewed the

irrigation line,' she said, by way of greeting, and adding, 'Again! And destroyed one of my pots: this one. You're looking for Maxie? Come in.'

Inside, Max was seated at the kitchen table, reading the Australian Financial Review with the deliberate stillness of someone who'd learned how to tune out both dogs and a wife with domestic disasters. He looked up, nodded once, and said, 'Rob,' and returned to reading.

Wager appeared behind him like a shadow. Tongue out, tail wagging, eyes bright, slobber everywhere around him, on the floor. Max lifted his head, as if having a sudden thought.

'Look, Wager,' addressing the dog, 'your friend has returned to take you away.' He then looked at me with his characteristic slanted, ever so slight sardonic smile.

'Well,' I said, patting the welcoming Wager. 'He looks healthy and, very happy,' and with that he then slobbered on me.

'Too healthy, and too happy,' Anne muttered, peeling off her gloves. 'He's demolished half the back hedge hunting for, who knows what? And he scared the living daylights out of Martha, our friend, the other day when they came to lunch. Wager slobbered on her from behind, and turning around, she thought he was a wolf. I doubt that they will ever come back!'

'She screamed,' Max added, still not looking up from his paper. 'Not a dignified scream either.'

Snippets of a Vet's Life

'And, Robert, she dropped her smoked salmon canape,' Anne said, like this was the greater offence, 'and then Wager ate it.'

Wager, as if on cue, sat down beside the kitchen bin and stared at it with hope.

'He's got a presence,' I offered.

'He's a bloody nuisance,' Max replied.

'He's Maxi's problem,' Anne added.

But they hadn't given him back.

That was the interesting part.

We moved to the sitting room, where Anne brought out a tray with coffee and shortbread that Wager clearly believed should be his. He tried, not so politely, to reach the edge of the tray with his nose.

Anne batted him away' 'Wager!' Max...do something! You know he's not allowed in here!'

'Perhaps Rob could take him away?' again that characteristic slightly sardonic look on his face.

'He's strong-willed,' I said. 'He clearly loves living here. Why would he want to leave?'

Max snorted.

'Leave! You gave him to us,' he said.

'Well... not quite. I made a suggestion.'

He folded the paper and leaned back in the chair.

'You said, 'Would you like to give a retired foxhound

a home?' I said, 'We'll see. Then he turned up.'

'And you let him in.'

'That doesn't mean I said yes.'

It was a point Max liked to make-not quite a joke, not quite a complaint. Just a quiet assertion that some things in life arrive without ever being officially accepted.

'If you had merely said no…and, let's be honest, he has a side to him that is engaging.'

'Engaging!' and Max noisily turned the newspaper to a new page.

Anne poured the coffee.

'He's clever, that Wager,' she said after a moment. 'Knows how to open the screen door. Got into the laundry basket the other day. Pulled out all my socks.'

'Just socks?' I asked.

She hesitated.

'And a few slips of paper.'

Max's eyes lifted from the paper now.

'Receipts,' she said.

I glanced at Max. He gave nothing away.

Anne enjoyed the occasional flutter; scratchies from the local IGA, and a quiet spin on the pokies now and then. She once explained it to me as "a bit of harmless fun," and I never questioned it.

Snippets of a Vet's Life

But Max? Max noticed things. He always did.

Wager had probably found one of her little tickets and trotted through the kitchen with it like he'd uncovered buried treasure.

Max and I had a quiet rhythm. I was still building up my vet business, and Max had become an unexpected sounding board. He never gave advice straight. He let me talk things through and then dropped a line or two that stuck.

I mentioned that I had recently hired somebody to help me with the office work.

'Her name's Joan. A bit older, but she seems very cheerful. Sings while she files.'

Max didn't look up from his coffee, but merely arched an eyebrow in response.

'Sings? Don't worry,' he said. 'Give her a month with your invoicing system. That'll shut her up.'

Another day, I told him I was thinking of doing more groundwork with tricky horses, behaviour stuff, and a bit of handling work.

Max stirred his coffee slowly and steadily.

'You have a natural talent with horses, but if you want my opinion?'

'I do...'

You remember that chestnut mare who taught you to fly backwards through a gate?'

I nodded. 'How could I forget?'

He took a sip, then said, 'Then don't.'

Anne, walking past with a laundry basket, chimed in.

'Max thinks he's wise because he reads financial papers. Truth is, he just likes the fold-out share tables.'

Max gave a long blink, as if to confirm the truth of it. Later, Max walked me out. The sun was low, and Wager trotted beside us, then bolted to the gate, woofed once, then returned.

'He's watchful,' Max said.

'Still got the hunter in him.'

Max nodded. He leaned on the gate and looked out across the paddocks.

'He's growing on you,' I said.

'I didn't say that.'

'You haven't thrown him out.'

He smiled then, just a little.

We stood in silence for a moment.

'I used to think the older I got, the less I'd want surprises,' he said. 'But sometimes you need something unpredictable. Something that won't do what it's told.'

'Like a foxhound.'

He nodded.

'Or a wife with a scratchie habit.'

Snippets of a Vet's Life

We both laughed, and Wager woofed again, once, sharp and clear. As I drove away, I glanced in the rear-view mirror. Max was still at the gate. Wager was sitting next to him, ears hanging, eyes forward, slobber drooling from his mouth. They seemed to be a team. He wasn't a good dog, not in the usual sense. But he was theirs now, whether they admitted it or not.

And Max, for all his grumbling, had let Wager into his life the same way he let people in, quietly, on his own terms, and rarely with a fuss. Anne always saw him as 'Max's dog. Maxi's problem.'

And Wager was content. He had found a home. And Max had a friend.

Rod Graham

29 – A DESPERATE NIGHT CALL

Late one Sunday night, while a storm blew about the Green Cottage, and the kitchen roof leaked, as it always did in a heavy downpour, the windows rattled and I heard a knock at the kitchen door. I was not expecting any visitors, and this seemed very late, I thought as I made my way to the door. There was a sudden gush of cold air, and a woman, her head covered against the storm, stumbled into the kitchen. I reached out and caught her before she could fall.

'Hi, Sue. What brings you here tonight? Is there a problem with one of the ponies?'

She had been a client of mine for a few years, but about a year earlier, her husband had left her. And I long suspected that one of the key disagreements in their relationship was the number of ponies she had acquired during their marriage and the drain it put on their finances.

The last time I saw Brian was when I treated one of her ponies for colic, and as often happens with colic, it was an 'all-nighter.' Luckily, the pony survived, but as it turned out, not the marriage.

I knew Brian felt caught by his wife's obsession with ponies. We were both walking Jiggles up and down the path, and periodically, the grey pony would throw himself on the ground in response to the sudden colicky pain. Brian was not naturally a talkative man, but on this occasion, he had a need. And there were numerous opportunities for us, as Sue had 15 ponies.

We walked up and down their garden path.

'You'd better save this one, Rob. I don't know what would happen if Jiggles were to die. He was a gift from her late Dad.'

'He's getting there, Brian. His heart rate has stabilised, so at least he is not getting worse,' and with that, Jiggles threw himself onto the ground. I reached down and slapped him.

The slap did it, and he jumped up. And we continued to walk him up and down the path.

'Rob, can I ask you something?'.

'Sure.'

'I'm at my wits' end, with her ponies. She bought another one last week, and when I try to discuss the increasing number of them with her, she closes me down by saying that I married her and her ponies.'

'Do you think things may change if you had a child?', I asked rather intrusively.

'Maybe, but with the state of our marriage, that is unlikely,' he paused, then continued, 'if you get where I'm coming from. I have always wanted children.'

And then suddenly he exploded in rage, 'I am SO SICK OF THIS,' and threw Jingle's lead in my general direction. Even Jiggles stopped his prancing and looked as Brian stormed away.

After a pause, I asked quietly, 'Are you OK, Brian?' His back was towards me, his shoulders slumped forward. His head was down. He looked like a broken man. In response, he held up his hand with its back towards me-the universal sign of a person needing space.

Jiggles again threw himself on the ground, and I slapped him on the flank to get him up. As I did so, I slipped and fell backwards into the rose garden. I let out an exclamation as I scrambled amongst the thorns. Brian heard the noise and ran over and grabbed the lead before the scrambling pony could run away.

'Thanks,' I said as I got to my feet, extricating myself from a rose branch. We resumed walking.

'She gets to love her ponies. They're almost like her children. They fill that need in her. But they don't fill that need for me. I don't hate the ponies; I'm just not into horses. And I don't know what to do,' he paused and then said, as we walked alongside each other with Jiggles between us, 'or perhaps I do.'

Snippets of a Vet's Life

I wasn't really surprised to hear that one day, after an argument with Sue, he went out to feed the ponies, which was his daily job. Having once fed them all, he got into his car, drove away, and didn't return. I never saw Brian again, but I did hear that he eventually remarried, moved to the inner city, and became a father.

And now Sue was unexpectedly at my door. I looked at her enquiringly as she stood just inside the kitchen door. Water dripped from her raincoat onto the kitchen floor.

'I got a call during the week from your office,' Sue said, paused, looked very uncomfortable, and went red in the face.

'Yes?' I said, somewhat confused.

'I'm here to pay the bill.' she said hesitantly.

I looked at her, wondering why she had chosen now, late at night, to knock on my door to talk about paying her account.

'Pay the bill?' I repeated her words, not quite sure what she meant by her presence at 11:30 pm. at my door on this stormy night. 'Come into the sitting room. Get warm.' Drops of water dripped from her raincoat onto the bare floor.

'I'm not sure how much your account is, Sue, so I'm at a bit of a loss on how to do this. Joan handles these matters at the office.'

'Yes, I got a call from her the other day about the

money I owe. I'm sorry, it's overdue. Even since Brian left. It's been a struggle.'

'I see. OK. How much do you want to pay?'

She looked away as I asked this question, and then she looked at me directly into my eyes.

'I was wondering if there might be another way that I could settle... my account?' She continued to look at me directly.

'Oh. What do you mean? I'm a bit confused.'

I was also, now I realise, just a bit dumb when it came to these situations. It took me a while, but eventually, the penny dropped... and then, I understood.

'Look, um. . . There is no need... uh. Just pay us when you can. I'll let Joan know that I have made a special arrangement with you. Take as long as you need. It is getting a bit late, do you think...'

'Yes. I best be off.' She looked relieved, and we both smiled nervously.

'Look, it's best if I walk you to your car. Can't be too careful these days.'

I was feeling very embarrassed, as I am sure she was. Later, I realised that for her to come to my door and make the offer, she must have been very distressed and perhaps at her wits' end as to what to do.

Horses, due to their very nature, size, and daily needs, are expensive to keep.

Snippets of a Vet's Life

My family always had one, and often two, horses when I was a child. Times were different then. We kept them in our backyard. The local Council (Shire) seemed little interested (at that time) in regulating backyard stables, and our area, in particular, had a plethora of them.

My Dad, as a mounted policeman, had introduced the family to the love and hatred of horses. And later, after leaving the police force, he worked as a lower-level manager of a sheep hides and skins business. My mother worked as a secretary for a small manufacturing firm. Not a lot of money. But as children, we did not 'want for a lot', but then again, we did not want much.

But we always, or so it seemed, had a pony in the backyard, and a racehorse, which my father trained.

I have occasionally wondered how we could afford them. Perhaps, we couldn't, which explained my mother's dislike of them, and perhaps was a part of the cause of their later separation and divorce. Again horses to blame for marital disharmony.

Rod Graham

30 – WHEN A MAN LOSES HIS MATE

I unconsciously listened as Joan, my secretary, took the call and made the appointment.

'That's a strange one,' she said after finishing the phone call. 'He's a new client and wants a second opinion on desexing his old dog.'

'Does he realise that we mostly do horses?'

'Yes. Apparently, he works on the wharf with George Matlock, and George recommended you, because he apparently said, that you are practical and you will tell him straight.'

So, I'm now 'practical', I thought. I have been called many things in my career, but this was the first time I was 'practical.' The appointment wasn't until the next day, and as I went about my work, I couldn't shake what had been asked of me: a second opinion on castrating an old dog. It was a strange request. Most male dogs were usually castrated at about six months of age, and I had not castrated one for a few years.

Snippets of a Vet's Life

I well remember that it was one of George's early morning visits, which had finally shown me the need for an office, and separate from my home.

***

George Matlock was a wharfie and loved his little pony, Tina. He was always concerned about Tina, and one early morning, on his way home from the night shift on the wharves, he had dropped in and knocked on my back door.

I was deeply asleep, but my slumber was rudely interrupted by the incessant knocking on the back door of the Green Cottage.

'Rob. Rob. Rob! Are you there?'

I made my way to the door, and just as I was about to open it, George yelled another 'Rob!' I opened the door, 'George. What's the problem?' It was about six o'clock in the morning.

'Oh, good. You are still in. I wanted to get to you before you left for the day.'

I tended to be a 'late' person, not an 'early' person. I also had sleep problems, so getting up early was very unusual.

'What's the problem?' I asked, fearing the worst.

'No major problem. I just wanted to make sure I could make an appointment today. Tina's got a cold, I think, and ....', but I interrupted him.

'Oh,' I said. 'Just one minute. I'll be back.'

With that, I closed the door, leaving George outside, and quietly walked across the kitchen. I silently opened the kitchen window, carefully climbed out of it and then ran across the adjacent paddock, inwardly yelling, 'I must get an office! I must get an office! I have lost my freedom! I can't get away!'

I stopped running about halfway across the paddock. I looked at my horse, Bos, who looked back at me with what I thought was a question, 'You OK? You're up early.'

He returned to eating grass. In his own way, Bos could sometimes be very understanding, or so I imagined.

I walked back toward the Green Cottage and climbed back through the window into the kitchen. I quietly closed the window and walked across the room. When I reopened the door, George still stood there. Feeling more composed, I asked, 'Now, George, what time would you like me to come out?'

Stress can manifest in various ways, and even I recognised that my reaction was a bit odd. I needed some distance between my home and my work, and be confident that I could turn off.

Eventually, I relocated the practice to the Old Cheese Factory, situated on the road leading into Coldstream. It was a long, white brick building with two levels. One side of the building had remained dormant and unused for several years, while the other side was occupied by a man who bred worms for anglers to purchase on their way to the streams of the distant ranges. The top level of the double-storied brick building adjoined the highway, and below, connected by internal stairs, was a large, double-storied work area that opened to an adjacent paddock. In this space, I was able to perform numerous operations on sedated horses using local anaesthetics and the occasional cat or dog.

***

I waited for George's friend to arrive for the 1 pm. appointment.

He was on time, and surprisingly, for the Yarra Valley of the '90s, he drove a clean, modern, baby blue Mercedes Coupe. He opened the passenger door, and a blue heeler dog struggled to get out of the car. He helped the dog up the small flight of stairs leading to the small landing and the office front door. I watched their slow progress through the window and opened the door for him and his dog as he reached the landing.

'Hi, I'm Rob, the vet. Please come in.'

He introduced himself.

'I believe you know George?'

'Yes. He recommended you as somebody who will tell me the truth.'

As he shook my hand, I noticed a roughness to his skin. He was short and stocky in build. This man had done heavy work, and his hands bore the marks of his past. His name was Eric, and he introduced me to his thin blue heeler dog, Roger.

The short walk from the car and up the stairs had exhausted Roger. Eric gently picked him up and carried him into the examination room. I gestured for Eric to sit on a chair, and I pulled another chair over and sat down facing him. Roger lay at his feet, and I could see that he was very frail, and he rested his head on his front paws.

'Now. How can I help you?'

'I want to know if I should castrate my dog. I went to a vet in town a while ago, and he wanted to castrate him. He was a young vet who didn't know what he was talking about. So I thought that I would see what a country vet thought. And George speaks highly of you. I trust George.'

I reflected that I was hardly a country vet, but I understood what he was talking about: I was trusted.

'Did you castrate him?'

'No! Of course not! Would you?' he asked rhetorically.

I looked at Roger. He was having slight trouble breathing. Each breath was quietly laboured.

'Eric. Why did the other vet suggest that you get him

castrated?' I had my suspicions about what the answer would be.

'There was a small lump near his bum, and he said that I HAD TO CASTRATE HIM,' and he emphasised the words.

I leaned over and gently lifted the dog's tail. There was a large lump to the left of Roger's anus. The diagnosis was obvious, even to a horse vet. Roger had a perianal adenoma, and the preferred treatment was castration. Once castrated, the tumour tends to shrink, and the issue is often resolved. However, if left untreated, especially with male hormone testosterone fuelling it, the tumour will grow and eventually spread to the lungs.

'Has Roger been losing weight lately, Eric?'

'Yep. I guess he's getting old. Like me. I was a shearer, and he always came with me on my trips.'

'Why didn't you get him castrated as the vet said to do?'

He looked at me aghast. Slowly shaking his head from one side to the other, he said, 'How could I? He's my mate! I wouldn't do that to my MATE!'

He was agitated, looking towards the closed door. He stood up. He looked around, then back at the door. Perhaps he was considering leaving. Then he took a deep breath and sat down.

I sat and waited until he regained control, retreating

into my professional mode: 'Best I have a look at him,'

I leaned down and listened to Roger's lungs; the sounds were muffled on the right side. I checked his gums. They were pale. He was probably anaemic, low in iron. His heart sounds were also muffled. There was something seriously wrong with his lungs. He coughed when I put slight pressure on his trachea with my fingers. I took his rectal temperature. He didn't move. It was subnormal.

'Eric,' I said. 'You realise he's in a bad way, don't you? I may be wrong, but I don't think he has long to live.'

I paused, conscious that I was being very direct. Was I being too brutal? Too direct. Did I have the right to destroy this man's hope in me? I continued, 'That's really why you are here, right?'

'I'm here because I want what is best for my mate. I want to save him. He's all I have. Can you save him? Can you fix him? I'm worried about him.'

Tears developed in his eyes. He looked embarrassed, and I looked away. I realised that telling Eric that he could have saved his dog if he had followed the advice of the previous vet would accomplish nothing. So why tell him, now? I quietly reflected that the young vet had probably not considered Eric's close emotional relationship with his dog. Suggesting 'castrating his mate' without explanation, listening, and discussion was an unintentional insult to Eric.

Snippets of a Vet's Life

After a few seconds, I looked back at Eric, and as I talked, I reached forward and caressed one of Roger's ears.

'I am sorry, but I don't think I can do a thing for him. The lump has probably spread to his lungs. See how he is having trouble breathing? Each breath is a struggle. I could take X-rays to confirm it, but just looking at how he is breathing. There is something very wrong.'

In a way, the profession had failed Eric and his canine mate, and now it was too late.

'All I can do now is gently put him out of his misery.'

Eric was looking at his dog as I talked, but after processing what I had just said to him, he lifted his head and looked directly at me.

'No. No. NO! I can't. I can't let you KILL my mate! He is all I have. I can't do that to him!'

He stopped and looked again at his dog and then, after a prolonged pause, continued,

'If you can't fix him, I guess I'll take him home and do my best to make him comfortable. Somebody suggested Rescue Remedy. It worked for their dog. Something… maybe. Or……'

'Rescue Remedy won't be enough, I am afraid. I could give you some painkilling drugs for him, perhaps cortisone for shrinkage? He will improve for awhile and then suddenly get worse.'

But before I could explain further, he stood up, shaking his head, and looking again at the closed door, indicated that we had finished.

'Eric, please listen. We have to do something...'

But he had stopped listening. He had lost faith in me. I had lost him. He wiped his eyes, leaned down, gently picked up his mate, and left the room.

Ignoring me, he paid his bill and carried his dog out the front door and down the stairs. He opened the door of the baby blue-coloured Mercedes and gently put his mate on the passenger seat. Once in the driver's seat, he backed the car out and drove away.

I never saw the blue Mercedes, Eric or his mate, Roger, again.

But I did run into George a few weeks later, as Tina, his pony, needed to be drenched for intestinal worms.

'George. Thanks for referring your friend with his dog. Any update?'

'He shot him not long after seeing you.'

I was somewhat shocked by the violence inherent in this revelation.

'Shot him?'

'Yep. As he said, it is what you do for a mate who is suffering.'

Snippets of a Vet's Life

31 – WHEN A BOY LOSES HIS MATE

I was on Rosemary's property to administer the horses' routine tetanus and strangle vaccinations. Even though he was old, Skip, like many kelpies, had enormous enthusiasm for visitors.

But on this day, Skip did not greet me.

'Still losing weight?' I asked.

'Yep. Not eating much now. Perhaps it's time?'

'Sounds like it.'

I was a horse veterinarian, but sometimes, in special situations, I would step back into the role of treating dogs and cats. Rosemary had asked if I could care for Skip. It was one of those special situations. Her son trusted me, and Skip was his dog, and Skip had a tumour in his abdomen.

This was before the easy access to the sophisticated diagnostic imaging that is now available. We had taken an X-ray some weeks earlier, and there was a faint suggestion of a lump on his spleen, but I could not be sure. I had warned the mother that the lump may have been a haemangiosarcoma and that sometimes such a tumour can start bleeding, the abdomen quickly fills with blood, and death can be relatively sudden.

But this did not happen in Skip's case. He had struggled on, and his energy gradually decreased.

It was time to 'do the right thing' and end Skip's life. The mother knew this. I knew this.

But did the boy know this?

He was about eight. About the age when the severe consequences of death begin to be understood by a child. And as Skip was his dog, should he be part of the process? Or should we just say that Skip had gone to the vet and wouldn't be coming back? Or should we say that Skip had run away?

Or…What?

Over the ensuing years, I have heard a variety of stories that parents have used in 'protecting' their young children from the death of an animal. And, sometimes, the 'children' are not so young. I have found that you can never predict how a family member will react to the imminent departure of a much loved pet. Even children with little contact for years with a family dog or cat sometimes need to be 'present.' If the child is overseas, they may request a lock of hair, an ink print of a paw, the collar, or some other keepsake.

For many, even if in life they were not close, ending a pet's life can be the last contact with their childhood. I usually follow the owner's wishes when it comes to ending a pet's life. However, there is one situation in which I advise caution: when a parent brings a dog or cat in for euthanasia without informing other family members, usually the children.

Rosemary had done, in my mind, the right thing. She had included her son in the process, even though, at eight years old, he was just on the cusp of understanding 'death.'

And Rosemary had brought the boy with her each time Skip came to see me.

I had discussed with the boy the seriousness of Skip's situation, how Skip felt unwell, and that Skip wasn't long for this world. And the boy had often listened with a solemn face to all I had said.

The boy loved his dog.

The following day, the three of us were in my makeshift examination room, with Skip on the table.

I looked out the window. The weather was bleak, rain pelted at the window, and cars wooshed to Yarra Glen or back towards Coldstream. Outside, life ebbed and flowed, and people were busy and went about their daily tasks, but inside, I was faced with the prospect of ending Skip's life.

'Tell me how you think Skip is feeling?'

'I don't think he is feeling very well.'

'Why do you say that?'

'Cause he doesn't play anymore. He just sits in his bed.'

'Is he eating?'

'No. I don't think so.'

'Do you think he is happy?'

'No.'

'What do you think we can do for Skip?'

I asked quietly, trusting that my questions had led him to the conclusion I wanted and that he would give me the answer I wanted.

'Can we make him better? I want to play with him again. I want him to run with me. Please, can you make him better?'

His pleading response surprised me. I had thought that he knew Skip was seriously unwell and, as he had been part of the process over the last few weeks, he would have realised that I could not make him 'better'. I thought he had understood.

He looked at his mother with tears in his eyes and held Skip close to his chest.

He looked back at me with pleading eyes.

'I can't make him better.' I said, pausing and then continued, 'I'm sorry. If I could, I would, but I can't.'

'But that means he will…die?'

'Yes,' I replied. 'And to let him die by not eating and not drinking would not be fair to him.'

Snippets of a Vet's Life

'I don't want him to die. I don't want him to suffer.'

His mother then spoke to him in a gentle, caring voice. We all need somebody to care at times like this. 'We have to let him go. You have to let him go. Skip is suffering. We need to do what Dr. Rob suggests,' she said, looking back at me.

I lifted Skip of the table, and onto the floor. I gently knelt and caressed Skip's neck, looking directly at the boy.

'What I want to do is inject, gently, into Skip's arm, a green-coloured drug. Only a tiny amount. A small injection. And you can hold Skip while I do this. After I have given him the injection, Skip will go floppy and fall asleep, and while he is sleeping, his heart will stop beating, and he will stop breathing, and he might even go to the toilet, so I will get you to hold him wrapped in a towel. He might then take a big breath; he might not. And then, after Skip's heart has stopped and he has stopped breathing, Skip will be dead. His life will have ended, and you have done something good for Skip. By making this choice, which I understand is very hard for you, to end his life, you have ended his suffering, which I can't fix...do you understand...what I am saying?'

The boy did not respond. Perhaps I had been too direct. I may have spoken too long and included too much detail.

He was quiet. He was crying. Skip sat in his arms.

Rosemary looked away. Perhaps she had tears in her eyes.

But I continued, 'I am going to leave the room now so that you can have a private time with Skip and your mother, and when you are ready to let Skip go, and when you can let me stop Skip's suffering, your mother will come out and get me, and I will return, and I will only then give Skip the injection. And Skip's life will end.' I paused and then asked, 'Do you now understand?'

He looked up at me and finally nodded. As I left the room, I gently closed the door. I could hear him cry, a gentle cry. After Skip was gone, the boy gently carried his body out of the room, out of the front door and down the stairs. The rain had stopped, and the sun was breaking through the clouds. Rosemary opened her car door and looked up at me, watching them through the window. She mouthed a 'thank you'

And then they were gone.

A Postscript

Over the years, we lost contact until recently, when I unexpectedly received the following note on my Facebook page from the mother, and with her permission, I shared her words:

'Many years ago, you put down my son's old (Kelpie). He wanted to be with (Skip). Rob, you gave my son time to say goodbye to his dog. You then came in and treated him with such gentle care. You described

all the procedures in step-by-step detail. I was so grateful. Thirty years have passed, and the memory is still vivid. Once again, thank you.

It is memories and thanks like this that bring tears to the vet's eyes.

Rod Graham

32 – AN UNEXPECTED VISITOR

The Green Cottage abutted the main road between Coldstream and Healesville. There was often a lot of traffic, especially during holiday weekends. The traffic sound was sometimes distracting, but after a few weeks of living in the cottage, I no longer noticed the intermittent noise of cars. In time the Green Cottage became my home.

But, there were few cars late at night, so to be woken up by a car stopping out the front and then roaring away with a skid, perhaps as it did a u-turn, was unusual.

I thought nothing of the interruption and rolled over to return to sleep. Then, I heard the sound of the front gate as the bottom scraped on the path, which brought me to full alert. I looked at the bedside clock, 2:45 am.

And as I was putting on shorts, there was a knock at the door. Perhaps somebody was lost or needed assistance, a client with an emergency or a stranger? I cautiously opened the door.

I was surprised that my late night visitor was the Matron's daughter.

Snippets of a Vet's Life

'Charlotte,' I said with surprise. And I noticed she was holding her shoes.

'Can I stay the night?'

I was somewhat taken aback by her question and stuttered an uncertain 'Yes' before continuing, 'I can make up the spare bed for you.'

'No need,' she said, giving me a look I had not seen in her eyes before. She walked past me and into my bedroom.

The following morning, I was roused from a heavy slumber by Charlotte, searching under the bed for something.

'Leaving? So early?' I said sleepily.

True to form, she ignored my question and then, after retrieving the lost article of clothing from under the bed, walked towards the bedroom door and said, as she was leaving, 'I thought you were different. But you're not! You're just like the others.'

She slammed the front door. And that was the last I saw of Charlotte.

What did she mean by suggesting I was just like the others?

About a week later, I saw the Matron in the supermarket. She was as ebullient as ever. She gushed general chitchat, and always polite, I listened. In a break in her conversation and feeling confused by Charlotte's recent visit, I asked, 'And how's Charlotte?'

Her mood instantly clouded over.

'Charlotte left after breaking up with her boyfriend about a week ago. She's living with her father now.'

Was her boyfriend driving the car that had been dropped off at the Green Cottage? I thought that was unlikely, but who then? And why? It was a mystery that remained unsolved.

'Oh. Her father? I think you told me that he was dying the night one of your horses had colic.'

'He's always dying. It's the way he draws Charlotte in.'

'Close by?'

'Yarck. He's not a nice man, but I don't want to speak about him.'

'OK. And Charlotte?'

'And she took the picture of my mother, off the wall without telling me. You may remember it.

'Why did she take the picture?' I asked, somewhat perplexed.

'Probably to sell. It's worth a small fortune now because of the artist. William Dobell. Her father is always trying to get money out of me, and that portrait is probably worth a few thousand dollars. I'm so angry with her!'

I think she was rarely a person who gave in to her emotions, but as she said the words, I could see that there were tears in her eyes. She looked away, and sniffed, and then back towards me, said, 'But she will return...I have her pony at least, and if she doesn't care for me, she at least cares for Pablo.'

I was unsure how to manage this emotional situation, so I merely said, 'When you do see her again, please give her my regards,' and turned to continue shopping.

As I walked off, she called out to me, 'Charlotte really did like you, Rob.'

I turned back to face her and asked, 'Did she?' I paused, as I considered her words. 'Did she really?'

'Yes!' she emphatically said, with a smile returning to her face, 'She did. She really did.'

My thoughts returned to the night one week earlier, when Charlotte had knocked on my front door., and left the following morning. I smiled back at the Matron, 'I do believe you, Matron. I really do. Thank you and goodbye.'

Rod Graham

33 – ACTING THE GOAT WITH A ROOSTER

My respect for horse dealers is genuine, though I know full well they are gloriously imperfect, much like the rest of us.

Imperfect? Certainly. So why do I respect them? Because they are often honestly dishonest, and I like honest people. I've met others, not horse dealers, who appear honest and trustworthy but turn out to be anything but. Those I call the "dishonestly honest", and I've never had much time for them.

Andy, the super car salesman, who had sold horses to the lottery winner, was one horse dealer, and Richie was another.

But Richie was a bit different to many horse dealers I met, in that he was mainly honest, and in time he became a good friend. He was also an honorary horse steward and, on this day, was in charge of entry into the arena at the Royal Melbourne Agricultural Show. We were both leaning over the arena gate, watching a jumping event, when he quietly announced, 'I have finished using your ute. If you want to get it at some point, you can.'

'OK,' I said, bemused, and then he added, 'And you owe me $1500.'

'So, Richie, so that I understand, for you to borrow my ute will cost me $1500. I'm feeling a bit confused. Can you explain why I owe you money even though I lent you the vehicle?'

I was confident that his answer would be interesting.

'Sure,' he explained, while still looking ahead, 'If you remember the state it was in when I borrowed it, the scratches to the paintwork and the few bumps in the body, I knew that you would get it repaired at some stage, so I organised it for you and saved you $1,500.'

'So... you did me a favour? By borrowing my ute.'

'Yep. But that's okay, because you are a friend. Otherwise, I would have passed the full cost on to anybody else.'

He gave me a sideways look as though what he had said was blatantly obvious. I could not fault his logic, but with Richie, the reality wasn't always as he described it. He might have arranged for the work to done for less than $1,500 and added a secret 'Richie service fee', just like the banks used to do. I would never know, but I always enjoyed our encounters, even though they often cost me money.

'OK. I'll pay you when I pick the ute up,' I said, unsure if I was being slightly defrauded. There was an uneasy silence as we watched the horse events in the arena until he asked quietly, 'You know anything about chooks?'

'No. Nothing. Not really. Why?'

'My wife has bought a rooster. She's mad about chooks. And she wants me to pick it up and pay for it.'

'Oh.' I absently replied, not sure where this was leading.

'Whenever I sell a horse, it often has to be checked by the vet. So, I think it is only fair that I get the rooster vet-checked. What do you think? '

I hesitated before I answered, still unsure where this was going.

Finally, I said, 'Yep.'

The Royal Show, combined with Richie, frequently brought out a naughty side in me, and this was one of those occasions, but recalling what we did then now leaves me feeling slightly embarrassed.

About an hour later, I was now dressed in a necktie and capturing the essence of a young, confident vet in my eyes. Richie and I entered the poultry pavilion and asked the attendant for a man by name. We were directed to the second row of poultry cages, where we found the old man sitting outside one of the cages. I could not help but notice the sag of skin under his old face, and combined with his thin face, he looked like, well...a rooster.

Behind him was a young, proud rooster in a cage.

'Hello. I'm Richie, and I am here to pay for a chook that my wife has selected.'

'Yes. Right you are,' and he dithered a bit as he stood up. 'This is the bird behind me,' and he indicated with an outstretched hand that he was expecting payment.

'Not so quick. This is my vet, and I brought him to check that the bird is healthy before I pay for it. OK?' said Richie.

He looked very startled at Richie and was clearly at a loss for words. I stepped up and announced, 'Hi, I'm Dr. Rob, but please call me Rob. Before I examine your bird, could I ask you a few questions? Is that OK with you?'

And I noticed that others in hearing range started to direct their attention towards us.

'Yes. I suppose. I have never had to do this before,' he hesitantly replied

'It won't take long. Just a few questions to start. Now Richie's wife wants to introduce your rooster to her girls, as she calls her hens.' I paused, and smiled at him, 'if you get my drift?'

He was an older man, and I could not take my eyes off his rooster-like jawline, as I continued, 'And that means..., and I'm not sure how to ask this, but do you think he is up to the job?'

'The job?' he queried.

'Yes. The job. You know what I mean?' and I nodded my head up and down.

He studied me, then his face lit up, and he nodded his head up and down.

'Oh, yes, the job! I understand. I don't really know,' and paused. 'How would I?'

'Well. It is probably an important part of why Richie's wife wants to buy a rooster. And as I am sure you will understand, if your rooster can't do the job,' and I winked at him, 'then well…do you see where I'm going?'

I noticed that the small crowd around us was gradually growing.

'I think he can. I think he's up to it,' the old man said, quietly leaning towards me. 'And he does make a rooster sound in the morning,' he added as evidence.

'OK. He sounds like a rooster?'

'Yes. Every morning.'

'Like… what sound?' I just could not resist.

'Cock-a-doodle doo,' he said quietly, bowing his head in my direction.

'What?' and I leaned towards him in response to his whispered answer.

'Cock-a-doodle-doo,' in a louder voice. I stood back. 'That's the sound he makes every morning,' and he repeated the sound, 'Cock-a-doodle-doo,' in an even louder voice, which had the effect of attracting more attention from the gathering crowd.

'Well, that sounds good. Let's move on to the next part,' I said, then asked, 'Can you get him out of the cage now? I just need to examine him.'

The old man retrieved the bird from the cage. He was obviously proud of his rooster as he held him in his arms. I took a stethoscope out of my pant's pocket, put the appropriate ends in my ears, and put the listening part on the left wall of the rooster's feathery chest. Beyond our small circle, more people gathered in the expanding small crowd of interested onlookers. I listened. And then I cocked my head and listened with a look of more serious intent.

'Um.'

Then I turned to the old man and said, 'Now, where he lives,' indicating Richie, 'there are foxes. Can your rooster fly?'

'I guess so. I've never seen him fly, but he does flap his wings, so I guess he could fly,' the old man said with an uncertain voice.

'OK. I need to test that. I want you to hold onto his legs, raise him above your head, and run up and down the aisle. Is that possible? '

And with that, I asked the crowd around us to make space so that the centre of the aisle was free.

'OK. Let's see how he flaps his wings. Start running.'

As instructed, the old man ran with the rooster above his head. The bird was flapping its wings as the man ran.

And as best as I could, I suppressed a smile, and Richie, a seasoned horse dealer, maintained a worried look. And even the old man had a slight smile on his face as he ran. Perhaps he was enjoying the attention of the growing crowd.

'That's good,' I said in an encouraging voice. 'Looking good. Now, can you just run the other way?'

And he did.

Again, the rooster wildly flapped its wings, only stopping when the old man returned to where we were standing. He then held the bird in his arms and cuddled the rooster against his own chest. I listened to the rooster's lungs and, again, his heart. I slowly shook my head.

'Interesting. Three heart sounds,' without adding, that this was normal for birds. 'Thank you for your assistance,' I said to the old man, and I turned to leave, and Richie turned to leave.

'When will you take the bird? And when will you pay me?' he asked.

'I'll be back later. Probably just before the Show finishes tonight, I have to consult with my vet and my wife,' Richie advised him.

And with that, we left the old man, his rooster, and the dispersing crowd.

'That was a bit of fun, Rob'

'I'm not sure, Richie. A bit naughty. I'm not sure we should have done that... and in particular... me.'

'Hey mate, loosen up!' he said with a smile as we left the poultry pavilion.

And although the old man had seemed to enjoy the attention, and perhaps even the rooster, the excitement, over the years I have occasionally reflected on my behaviour.

It was a lesson learnt.

From then on, this encounter established a guiding rule for my professional behaviour: never to make fun of clients at their expense.

As we walked, I had another slightly worrying thought.

'I hope the Vet Board doesn't hear of it.'

And it was only years later that I learnt that when Richie returned, later that day, to pay for the rooster, he negotiated a lower price because it had a 'dodgy heart'.

34 – LUCY'S LAST LIGHT

When Max McClintock rang, it was a wet, cold Thursday morning in Spring, and ankle-deep in mud, I was removing a retained afterbirth from a mare. I had recently installed, at great expense, a mobile phone in my car. I cleaned my arm of lubricant and ran to the car.

'Rob,' he said. 'Lucy's eye is crook. She's holding it shut, and I can't get near her with a torch or a biscuit.'

'Is it swollen?'

'No. Just weeping. And she's not herself. Didn't finish her hay, wouldn't walk up to the gate this morning.'

'Alright. I'll be there this arvo.'

'Appreciate it.'

He hung up without a goodbye. Max, as I have said before, was never one for unnecessary words.

Apart from his wife, Anne, he had one other love in his life. Lucy was a thick-set, plain-faced Quarter Horse brown mare, gentle and smart. The sort of horse that always knew where the gate was and never spooked at shadows. She'd been with Max longer than most of his horse agister clients. Lucy was already a resident when I began working as a veterinarian for Max.

When I arrived, Lucy was standing under the big gum in the corner of the paddock, head lowered. Her left eye was squeezed shut, and tears ran down the side of her face. She turned her head slightly as I approached, but didn't shy away.

'Looks painful, Max,' I murmured, reaching for her halter.

Max stood nearby, arms crossed, frowning and obviously concerned.

'I thought it might've been a stick or something, but I've checked the paddock. Nothing obvious, and there are no low-lying branches.'

I pried the eye open gently. A faint bluish haze was visible over the cornea. The pupil was constricted and unresponsive to my little pen torch. There were signs of pain, but no pus or foreign body.

'Looks like uveitis,' I said.

'Is that bad?'

'It's inflammation inside the eye. It can be painful. Usually from trauma, infection, or something systemic. Hard to say at this point. It could be a knock. Trauma to an eye usually explains this appearance.'

'Can she go blind?'

'Not usually. Not if we treat it early and keep it under control.'

I pulled out atropine drops to dilate the pupil, a tube of steroid ointment, and a few sachets of bute, a cheap pain-relieving and anti-inflammatory drug, in powder form for oral, administration.

'Twice a day with the ointment. The atropine is once daily. And feed her this powder for the pain and inflammation. I'm expecting an uneventful recovery, but if it gets worse, just give me a call.'

Max took the supplies like I'd handed him a baby. 'She won't like it. She's a bit funny about things in her food. A bit like Anne in that regard.'

'Mix the powder molasses, and put that in her food.'

'We'll see young veterinary.'

Max, in line with many of my clients, had been watching All Creatures Great and Small on television, and had started calling me his variation on the word "viterinary", a term the farmers used in the tales of a young Yorkshire vet. I saw it as a term of endearment and respect.

Lucy improved over the weekend, as I had anticipated. Max reported she was brighter, walking better, and eating normally again. I told myself we'd nipped it, whatever it was, in the bud.

Then came Tuesday.

'Rob,' Max said on the phone. 'It's back. Worse. And

it's in the other eye now. And she's off her food.'

When I arrived, Lucy was pacing the fence line, bumping gently into the rails as she went. Both eyes were now affected, half-shut, hazy, dripping. Her confidence was gone. Her ears flicked constantly. She startled when I touched her neck.

'This isn't a knock,' I said. 'This is something bigger. Looks like something medical'.

'Like what?'

'I don't know.'

I said it out loud, surprising myself with the honesty. I'd seen uveitis before, sometimes in cats, post-vaccination, but never this severe, never in both eyes, and never in a horse. Ever. I was at a loss. I updated the treatment. More atropine, systemic steroids this time, more potent anti-inflammatories, but I was starting to feel out of my depth.

As I packed my kit, Max gestured at the feed shed.

'By the way, rats are back. Big ones.'

'Wager's not helping?'

'Wager! He is, of course, absolutely useless as a rat catcher. I think he made friends with one of them. Brought it into the laundry. I wouldn't be surprised if he slept beside it. Anne wasn't pleased, if you get my drift.'

'Sounds like he has become a pacifist living here.'

'Well. Anne is certainly not that! And that Wager you dumped on us is a waste of space.'

'Ah. I see that you have a hidden affection for him. Max. Sounds like you need a cat.'

'We have one, but it appears to be missing in action. And, my good friend, I suspect Wager.'

That night, I sat down at the kitchen table with the fat veterinary reference manual I rarely opened now, and stared at the "Uv" section in the index.

Equine recurrent uveitis, commonly seen in appaloosa and warm bloods horses often of idiopathic origin, may be associated with systemic infections or immune-mediated triggers.

I hated that word, idiopathic. Why didn't they just say 'of unknown cause'? The book was of no help.

I rang Peter, an older vet who had been in the Yarra Valley for years. He was semi-retired, the kind of vet who had a chronic cough, and whom the clients loved; and for some, he was the oracle. He must have been an excellent student years earlier because he told me one day that he kept folders of all his case notes like gospel. I kept them in my head, like most horse vets did in those times.

'Bilateral uveitis?' he said. 'Not a common one. Any signs of infection?'

'Nothing obvious. No fever, no nasal discharge. Just the eyes.'

Snippets of a Vet's Life

'Exposure to rats?' The question came out of the blue and surprised me.

'Rat? Everywhere. You could say the owner could rent them out.'

Peter paused. 'Check for leptospirosis. I first saw it a few years ago, in a cow. It was diagnosed after we put it down. The government vets were very interested, and they did all the testing. Not sure how they got the answer, but they were sure: lepto.'

'But. In a horse? Do you know? Any idea?'

'Probably. Certainly, in pigs, sheep, and goats, from what I recall. I think I read somewhere that it can affect dogs, and to a lesser extent, cats.'

I was secretly amazed at the breadth of his knowledge. He was a real resource, and I understood why he was popular with farmers.

'From what I remember. I think the Agriculture Department issued a notice to vets at some point. Those notices are handy. You should sign up for them. Under-diagnosed. Lepto can cause uveitis, at least in cows. Probably horses as well. It's not in the textbooks yet, but I've seen it a couple of times. Usually both eyes, delayed onset, and no other signs. Usually after a warm spell and some standing water.'

'Bloody hell, Peter,' I said. 'I wouldn't have thought of that in a hundred years.'

'But that's why you called! Glad to help. And Rob, I

want to thank you for the various times you've helped me when this cough has got the worst of me.'

Again, I reflected that I was part of a collegiate profession, even though we competed for clients.

Back at Max's, I explained what I'd learned, and from whom.

'Leptospirosis?' he repeated. 'From rats?'

'Yes. From their urine. It can get into feed, water, or anywhere they've passed through. Horses pick it up without symptoms, and weeks later, the eyes can react.'

Max didn't say anything for a while.

Then, quietly: 'So this was preventable, or treatable?'

'Possibly. But we couldn't have known. Even if we'd guessed, there was no easy test to confirm it. Still isn't, really, unless we aspirate fluid from the eye.'

He nodded. 'Wouldn't be fair on her.'

'No.'

(Nowadays, a simple blood test will diagnose the disease in ten minutes.)

Despite our best efforts, Lucy's vision continued to deteriorate. She started walking into posts. She spooked at nothing. Her confidence was gone. Max built a little corral near the house to keep her safe, but she circled it nervously, ears flicking, tail swishing in confusion.

Snippets of a Vet's Life

Then one morning, he rang me, his voice flat.

'She walked into the trough. Cut herself up. I think she's scared. It's not fair. I think it's time'

'I'll come now.' I had been expecting the call.

We led her to the base of the old gum tree. I had passed this tree many times over the years. The sun was warm, and we were surrounded by silence, broken only by the occasional rustling of the leaves above.

He held her gently, and to my surprise, rested his head against her neck. He murmured something. Soft, private words that I couldn't quite hear. Maybe they were goodbyes. Maybe just gratitude. And once again, I was reminded that there's no right script for saying farewell to a companion you've loved. It's never easy. It's never tidy. It's just what it is. Hard. He lifted his head and looked at me.

'Ready, Max?'

'Ready as much as you can be in this situation.'

'Here's what I plan to do. First, I'll administer a tranquilliser into her jugular vein in her neck. That will help her relax. Then, I'll insert a catheter or large-bore needle into the same vein to establish a clear line into her bloodstream. Once you give me the nod, I'll connect a 20ml syringe filled with the drug to the catheter and inject it quickly. Next, I'll remove that syringe, attach the next full one, and repeat the process. There are five in total. I need you to pass me each syringe as I finish with one. Can you do that?'

'Yes. Why does it have to be done so fast?'

'So she drops quickly, without struggling or panicking, as she begins to lose her footing. The drug I'm using is a very strong anaesthetic agent. It's like hitting the brain all at once, so she goes down quickly and peacefully, without fear or resistance.

I sedated her gently, stroked her neck, and talked to her softly.

I looked at Max.

'Ready?'

'Yep. Let's do it.'

I connected the syringe and rapidly injected the drug, syringe after syringe, and as I injected the last dose of the drug, she folded slowly, gracefully, like a curtain drawn at the end of a play.

There was no struggle. As planned, she quietly slumped onto her knees, then rolled onto the ground. Gone. I waited for a final agonal breath, but there was none. She was dead.

'Max. This may sound unusual, but if you are able, I suggest placing your hand on her neck. Just pat her.'

He looked at me, and on his face was an unsaid question, 'Are you for real?'

'Trust me. Just do it.'

Snippets of a Vet's Life

He did. And his look of grief was replaced with a look of quiet acceptance.

'She really has gone. Just the body is left. I see what you mean. Gone.'

We were both quiet and in the moment.

'You know, viterinary, the body is really a mere vessel for the memories. And that's why you got me to touch her. The vessel may have gone, but not the memories.'

'Max. I have never heard it expressed so well before. I think you are exactly right. And by making the hard choice, to end her life, in a way, you have given her your last gift, to end her suffering, in return for all the years of what she has given you.'

He looked at me with a gentle, knowing smile, and I believe there were tears before he looked away.

While I tidied up and made good to leave, I asked, 'Any questions?'

'Nah. Just give me a hand with her.'

Without either of us saying any more, we rolled her dead body into a hole dug earlier by a neighbour with a backhoe.

'Thanks, veterinary', (he reverted to more customary pronunciation).

He turned and walked back towards the house alone.

About a week later, I had to make a routine call back to Max's property.

'So that's the first time you've seen this lepto thing?'

'First time I've recognised it,' I said. 'Might have missed it before.'

'Can't win them all, veterinary,' was all he said.

Some cases settle into your memory not because they were loud or tragic, but because they quietly altered something in you. Lucy's case was like that. She wasn't the sickest horse I'd ever treated, or the most dramatic, but she was the first I watched go blind from leptospirosis. And the truth is, I didn't see it coming. I didn't even know where to look. It taught me that being a vet doesn't mean having all the answers; it means knowing when to ask for help.

And Max? He faced it all with quiet grace. He never raised his voice, never pointed a finger. He just did what had to be done and then just got on. Maybe that's why it stays with me. Maybe that's why the memory of losing Lucy still lingers. Maybe.

35 – THE STITCH UP AND THE SECRET

Let me call him Hans. I was sound asleep one night when my bedside phone rang. I lifted the receiver, knowing that it often meant losing two or three hours of rest.

'Rob, one of my agister's horses has gone through a fence in this storm, and she wants you to stitch up the leg.'

He named the horse's owner, and after hearing the extent of the horse's injury, I knew that I had to go.

I didn't know much about Han's backstory. I knew he had been teaching dressage for many years. He was coming to the end of his career. He was gradually falling out of favour, but he still had some long-term clients, one of whom had recommended me. I wasn't Hans' preferred vet, but our mutual client had sung my praises for repairing cuts on horses' legs, so he called, and I went.

I drove in the rain to the office, picked up some surgical instruments, and travelled along the highway in the dead of night, mostly alone on the wet road.

He was classically European. He stood very upright, even though I estimated that he must have been in his late 70s. He had a weathered face and a small grey moustache. He greeted me with a heavy Austrian accent, 'Ah! Rob! Thank you for coming out on such a night.'

He led me to the paddock and the shed in the corner of the horse's paddock by torchlight. The rain was starting to fall again, and we caught the horse and made the cover of the shed just before the next downpour.

While Hans held the torch and the horse's lead, I did my best to support the horse's leg as I tried to perform an adequate repair to its wounded leg. Meanwhile, a strong wind was lifting part of the shed's roof, causing water to drip down on me. With the wind, the horse would shy and stamp its leg, forcing me to start again. Sterility is a wonderful concept, but it's not always achievable in a storm. Without the judicious use of penicillin, many a stitch-up would end up in an infected mess a few days later.

These situations, where one person, in a storm, is restraining a nervous horse, and the other is attempting to stitch a wound on a leg, are made for conversation… or swearing. Hans and I chatted about many now-forgotten topics.

And as I stitched, he told me harmless stories about people we both knew and finally, the job was finished.

Snippets of a Vet's Life

'Would you like some fine Austrian coffee to warm you up before you go?' he asked.

While I had coffee, he had a few whiskeys, and his conversation flowed. I mostly listened. I had not been in his house before, and as he chatted, I noticed pictures on his wall of the Spanish Riding School in Vienna.

'Did you ride there?' I asked.

'Yes, when I was much younger. For a while, until the war.'

I knew that during the Second World War, the famous white Lipizzaner mares were moved to Hostau in Czechoslovakia, and I asked,

'Did you go with them to the country?'

'No,' he replied. 'I wasn't allowed. We were technically in the army, and many from the school became officers.'

I quietly considered what he had said.

'So...Hans...you would have been on the other side?'

'Yes... Of course, Rob. Is that a problem?'

'No,' not sure what to say next. He was the first Axis soldier I'd met, and as such, had been under the control of the German army. There was an uncomfortable silence in the room.

'I'll let you in on a secret.'

He was becoming more loquacious as the whisky had its effect.

'I was in the SS.'

'The SS. No way,' I said incredulously, somewhat unsure how to continue. 'You do mean the German SS?'

The SS (Schutzstaffel) was the elite guard of the Nazi regime and a virtual state within the Third Reich, and often inflicted cruel punishments or death on their prisoners.

'Yes. I had no choice. I was an officer,' he said softly, as if testing my reaction.

'No choice?'

'Yes, no choice,' he repeated, smiling at me, and I felt uncomfortable. I looked at the clock. 2:00 am

'Well, Hans. It is getting late. Thank you for the coffee; I think it is time I head home,' and I made my way to the door.

'Have I upset you?' and he stumbled a bit as he got up from the table.

'Perhaps I have said too much. Yes?'

'No. Very interesting, but I must go. It is just getting late. I have a long trip home.'

In truth, I wasn't sure what to say. I had read a lot about the Second World War, and I knew about the SS and their brutality. I was unsure if what he was telling me was entirely the truth.

Snippets of a Vet's Life

To this day, I still don't know. But why would anybody profess to be a member of the SS? Even as a poor-taste joke. Was he trying to shock a young vet? Why did he tell me? I realised he had revealed a dangerous secret that could have ended his career in the Yarra Valley if others found out. Why did he trust me with this secret? Throughout my career, I became the bearer of many people's secrets and shared countless private moments.

This was one of them, one stormy, wet night, a long time ago.

36 – THE DRUNK NEIGHBOUR

Some moments forever bring a smile to a vet's face, and this is one of them.

There was an urgent knock at the clinic door. I opened it to find an older man I barely knew, except in passing. He was standing at the top of the stairs and holding a squirming West Highland Terrier in his arms. The dog wasn't just wriggling, he was lurching, his little legs flailing as if gravity had forgotten how to work correctly.

'Ah, good! You're in. Sorry to bother you, Rob, but my dog's acting strange. He's drunk!'

I blinked. I'd seen dogs with odd neurological signs, seizures, poisonings, even strokes, but rarely did owners sum it up quite so plainly.

'Come in. This way.'

I led him to the exam room. He followed awkwardly, arms full of a white terrier and his face full of concern.

The man was Gerald, the worm-farm owner and my neighbour from next door. We had a relationship where we would nod at each other as we passed, instead of

Snippets of a Vet's Life

talking. He ran a bait business behind the old Cheese Factory, breeding live worms for passing anglers heading to the high country. He kept to himself. So did I. We had separate entrances and did not need to chat after that brief meeting when I started working out of the old Cheese Factory.

'He's been a bit off lately,' he said, gently placing the dog on the table. 'He stumbles around, stares at the walls. Then he's better for a few days. Then it's back again. Sometimes he has the squirts and goes off his food, but only for a few days. But he's never been this bad.'

The Westie, called Benji, swayed on his feet. His pupils reacted slowly. His head bobbed as if tracking something invisible. He did look drunk.

'Any chance he has been drinking beer or alcohol…'

'Nah. I'm a teetotaller. Don't drink. No alcohol on the premises or at home.'

I ran my hands over Benji. No heat. No pain. No injury. Just a vague, woozy dog who looked like he'd wandered out of a pub after a long session. I tested his reflexes. Checked his ears. Asked about his diet, trauma, and toxins. Nothing quite added up.

'Have you noticed anything else odd?'

'His breath's been strange. Sour. And sometimes he smells like… damp bread.'

That made me stop. I sat at my desk while Benji swayed at his owner's feet.

Mentally, I wandered through the list of weird and wonderful possibilities. Inner ear? No. Seizures? Too typical. Toxin? Maybe. Snakebite? But he was too active. Time to hit the books or lecture notes.

'Gerald. I must admit, this is unusual. Wait a minute while I look up a textbook or two. OK?'

'Sure. Whatever it takes. I'm worried.'

I spun my chair and scanned the bookshelf. I'd kept one of my old vet school volumes, a heavy red reference on obscure poisonings and environmental hazards. I flipped through the section on toxins.

Then a heading caught my eye: Fermentation By-Products-Ethanol Exposure in Companion Animals.

I read it once.

'Hello. This may be what we are dealing with,' I announced.

Then again, I read and my eyes narrowed as I took in what it revealed:

Low-grade ethanol. Produced by microbial fermentation. Often seen in home brewing, worm farms, compost…worm farms!

I turned back to Gerald.

'What exactly do you keep in those worm beds of yours?'

Snippets of a Vet's Life

He shrugged.

'Veggie scraps. Bread. Some brewery mash the pub gives away. The worms love it.'

'And Benji?'

'He goes with me everywhere. Sleeps in the shed. Fell into a tub last week. Covered in muck.'

That was it! I felt secretly proud of myself, secure in my belief that I knew the answer.

'He's not sick. He's not dying. He's drunk. Just like you said.'

'What?'

'Worm farms can ferment, especially when you add grains or mash. They heat up, break down, and produce small amounts of ethanol and other waste products. If he's licking the compost or licking it off himself, he's absorbing enough to get intoxicated, especially for a dog his size.'

Gerald stared at me.

'You're telling me... the worm farm got him pissed? He does eat some of the bits that fall on the floor when I'm getting out worms for a customer. So that's it? I can't wait until I tell the boys at golf. You certain?'

'Fairly. We may never know for sure, but I'd stop Benji from eating any leftover worm-farm stuff if I were you. It's low-grade exposure, but the symptoms fit: wobbly gait, strange behaviour, intermittent signs, and it wears off after a few hours, or even a day or two.'

He looked down at Benji, now curled peacefully on the table with one ear twitching.

'What do I do?'

'Let him sleep. He may get the runs, but eventually he'll come out of it. IF he starts vomiting, let me know, but I think he is going to be OK. I'd fence off the worm beds. Hose him off properly if he falls in again. And maybe cut back on the brewery mash. Even to me, it smells delicious, and probably to Benji too.'

Gerald chuckled despite himself.

'Poor bugger. I thought he was losing his mind.'

I smiled, still holding the textbook in my lap.

'Turns out you were right all along. He was drunk.'

Snippets of a Vet's Life

37 – THE PURVEYOR OF DREAMS

Horse dealers are among the best salesmen I have ever met, and I have dealt with many of them.

They inherently would find out what it was you wanted to buy, create a story, sometimes true, sometimes not so true, about the horse that they wanted to sell you, and then, appearing to believe their own story, they would 'honestly' sell you what you wanted to buy.

One dealer, in particular, was exceptionally skilled at reading people. He had about sixty horses in a paddock on the edge of the city. He would run various advertisements in the city papers each week, offering his horses for sale.

Whether the horses, as advertised, ever existed was always a moot point. In the end, it did not matter because when a prospective buyer arrived at his paddock, he would say to them,

'There are sixty horses out there. Go out and sell yourself one. Then come back and we will talk.'

I always thought this was an interesting way to sell something. It was also very efficient.

The prospective new owner would find a horse that appealed to them, return to the dealer, and then negotiate a price, with the dealer having the advantage of knowing they now wanted the horse. I suspect that the price then went up.

This man was not formally trained in economic theory, but he knew the basics of sales. Most purchasers buy what they want instead of what they need. They also buy images and dreams. And the horse dealer was a master at creating dreams and possibilities, then selling them to you.

This was brought home to me one day when I was called to a stable just outside of Coldstream.

Josie, a new client, asked me to check her horse's eye. I could see that the horse was a bit skittish, so I parked my car slightly away from them in an effort not to startle it. She was concerned about the eye because she had recently purchased the horse from a local horse dealer.

It was the first horse she had bought, and she was worried that she might have purchased a horse with a 'problem.' The right eye was slightly closed, and as I approached the horse to examine it, the horse shied back away from me. And as it attempted to do this, one of its hind legs snapped up, almost hitting its abdomen. Then, as the leg returned to the ground, the other leg did the same.

Snippets of a Vet's Life

I was expecting Josie to be alarmed by this movement, but instead, she had a smile on her face.

'That's interesting,' I said, but knowing that the horse had stringhalt, an involuntary reflex movement of the hind legs caused by nerve damage and frequently seen in horses grazing on dandelions and some other pasture weeds.

Sometimes, the condition would self-correct, but it could take months, and sometimes, the horse needed surgery. Over the years, I have operated on many horses in an attempt to correct the problem, but not always successfully.

'Yes,' she said, adding, 'I'm lucky that I got him, but it cost me extra.'

'Lucky in what way?' I was truly intrigued.

'Well. I actually wasn't going to buy a horse. I went with a friend a few weeks ago, and while walking around the dealer's paddock looking at horses, I saw this one and noticed the hind leg movement. I secretly wanted a Tennessee Walking horse, but never thought I would be able to have one or afford one. I always thought they walked with exaggerated front leg action, but when I spoke to the dealer, he explained that this horse was one of the rarer ones with exaggerated hind limb action.'

'Did he?' I said, more intrigued, thinking that this was truly a sales angle I had never heard before!

'The dealer mentioned that many people were keen on buying this horse and that if I wanted him, I should purchase him right then and there, so I did.'

'How long ago?'

'About a week, but I am now worried about his eye.'

I did what she wanted and examined the eye. It had a mild case of conjunctivitis and would be better in a few days with simple treatment. While I was attending to the horse's eye, I had time to think.

She had bought a horse that was precious to her, paying extra for its perceived rarity. She wasn't seeking my opinion on her purchase but rather on the horse's eye. I also realised that once her story got out to her friends and she started taking the horse out on rides, she would suffer ridicule and mockery. Nothing was more certain.

It was an ethical dilemma for the young vet.

'Josie,' I said. 'I can understand why you think you have purchased a Tennessee Walking Horse. As far as I know, they always have an exaggerated front-leg gait. Never the hind legs'

She looked at me, alarmed.

'I don't think this is one of them. I think your horse has a condition called stringhalt,' and I explained what that was.

She was horrified and wanted to know what to do about it.

Snippets of a Vet's Life

'Well,' I said, 'that is an interesting question. You bought the horse a week ago?'

'Yes.'

'Well, you could try going back to the horse dealer and see what he can do. I'm not sure that he will do anything because I think he has sold you a dud horse, and too much time has passed.' I added, 'You may have to get legal advice.'

Josie called me a few days later and reported that the eye was much better, and added that she had been in contact with the horse dealer and had told him what I had said about her new horse. But the horse dealer had said that because I was young and inexperienced, I did not know what I was talking about, but then added that because of the doubt I had raised, he was 'very sympathetic', but he could not give her the money back. But, because she was young and he liked her, he told her that he would exchange the horse for another.

'That's good, ' I said, 'but I strongly suggest that you take a vet with you this time and get the new horse checked.'

I wasn't sure that was exactly what the horse dealer had said about me, but I was pleased that Josie would at least get some value for her money. As it turned out, she had used another horse vet, and I lost her as a client, which left me a bit surprised. And if I was honest, deflated.

As my older veterinary colleague, Gerald, once said, owners tend to rotate through horse vets in a 4 to 5 year cycle.

About five years later, I met Josie again. She was upset with her previous vet. Apparently, it had something to do with his 'outrageous bill,' and she had decided to call me because, as she told me, she had always trusted me after our previous encounter. And I could at least get an update on our previous encounter with the horse that had stringhalt.

As the dealer had promised, he took the horse with stringhalt back and then promptly sold her a dressage horse that had 'nearly gone to the Olympics, but for having colic on the day the Australian Olympic team was due to leave the country.'

The new horse had cost her about $1000 extra because of the Olympic connection, but she had been happy with it, even though she had never been able to get it up to a high standard in dressage because of her lack of ability.

'Good,' I said. 'I'm happy that it worked out for you.'

I then asked, already knowing the answer, 'Did you take my advice and get a vet to check out the new horse?'

'I would have used you because I trusted you, but I knew that you didn't like dressage horses, and you didn't know much about them, so I called the other vet. And he was older.'

Snippets of a Vet's Life

'Oh. That's interesting. Who told you that I didn't like dressage horses and didn't know much about them?'

'The horse dealer.'

38 – A COLLEAGUE AND A COW IN NEED

He had called early Sunday morning to explain that the family's cow was down and having trouble calving.

'There's one leg sticking out, but nothing is happening. I think she needs help. I think she has been like that for a while.'

'I'm not sure that you have called the right vet. I don't tend to treat cows. Mostly horses. Perhaps you should give...' I paused and was about to give him my previous boss's contact details when he interrupted me.

'Actually, it was Dr Doug who suggested I give you a call. He's a bit unwell.

Good enough. Doug was reaching out for help.

Even though I had left the world of being a general vet, horse owners would occasionally ask me to attend to other animals. Typically, it would be in the form of, 'While you are here, could you look at Penny, our goat,' or 'If you have a minute, before you go, could you just look at Rosemary, our cat?' And frequently, Penny would still be in the paddock, and Rosemary, nowhere to be found.

Snippets of a Vet's Life

But this was slightly different.

Occasionally, I was called back to my past life when one of my colleagues asked for help. It has always been a collaborative profession. This was one of those situations-a colleague in need, to help with an animal in need.

'Sure. Glad to help you,' I replied.

On the way, I noticed that the orchards had lost their leaves, and in parts, Parslow's Creek was flooding low-lying pastures. A recent storm had left small branches on the road, so I took more care in driving.

I enjoyed winter, even though it meant sometimes working in the wet and muddy conditions. From my past job with Doug, I learnt that Autumn calvings were the norm in the area, but sometimes a cow calved in early winter. Nothing else could be done but to strip down and help, no matter the state of the weather.

His directions to their small farm were excellent. As I pulled up outside the house, rain started to fall. Jerry Brown stood on the verandah, holding an umbrella. I introduced myself and shook his hand.

'I'm sorry, but she's out the back still, not in a shed. I thought she had a few more days; otherwise, I would have put her in a shed before calving. But...' He looked up at the clouds. 'I do have an umbrella, which we can use.'

'That's OK, Jerry. Let's see her. Don't worry about the rain. The main thing is that we help her. Show me the way.' I was resigned to getting wet and, if she were down, lying in the mud.

The cow sat on her chest in a low dip in the ground next to a wire fence. As I walked towards her, she attempted to get up but was unsuccessful and slumped back down. A calf's foot protruded from under her muddied tail.

'How long do you think she's been like this, Jerry?'

'Don't know. We went to church, and I found her when we returned. Sorry.'

'That's OK. Nothing to be sorry about. These things happen. Do you happen to have a tarp that I could put behind her so I can lie down and keep the situation as clean as possible? And some hot water…in a bucket?'

Even though it was cold, I stripped down to only my pants. My top was bare. I shivered in the driving rain. Jerry held the umbrella over me as I slathered obstetrical lubricant on my right arm. Then, lying on my side and behind the cow, I gently inserted my arm into the birth canal, following the exposed calf's leg inward.

The cow, perhaps in response to the pressure of my arm, had a contraction that clamped down around it. I waited. There was nothing else to do. When it passed, I pushed deeper, my fingertips guiding me. Another contraction, but weaker this time.

Snippets of a Vet's Life

In a normal birth, a calf presents with the front feet first and the head between the knees and shoulders. Any other presentation signals trouble.

However, my exploring hand soon reached the issue. The exposed foot was part of a front leg, but the calf's head was turned back, and the other leg was trapped.

Even though I hadn't faced this exact situation before, I knew what to do. As a student, I had been trained for it.

People sometimes say vets have it harder than doctors because we deal with so many species. It's not quite true. We learn the principles and apply them. For instance, the structure of a pig's abdomen is similar to that of a human's. That of a cat and a dog is almost the same. However, we must always adapt to the situation at hand, applying the principles learned as students.

And we ask questions differently, too. If someone collapses on a train, a doctor will attempt to rouse the patient in an attempt to talk to them. A vet will speak to the witnesses. That's how we work. By drawing out the useful detail others miss. As one of my clients had commented, a good vet has to have the skills of Sherlock Holmes.

Another contraction passed. I worked my arm deeper until I could get behind the calf's jaw, cupping its nose. Gently, I pushed the head back, then guided it into the birth canal. Meanwhile, the rain continued. Jerry tried to shelter me, but I was soaked through. The only warm part of me was my arm inside the cow.

Now that the head was aligned, I reached further and freed the trapped front leg, guiding it up beside the other.

I removed my arm and pumped more lubricant into her. Then I carefully fitted two eye hooks into the bony edge of each eye socket, not the eyes.

'Now, Jerry, pull gently, downwards, and in the direction of her hooves. The birth canal curves downward. Got it?'

'Got it,' he said, and he pulled gently, and I guided the head and legs through the birth canal.

Then, with a soft plop, the calf slid out. The calf wasn't breathing. I began chest compressions. At the same time, the cow rose, and the steam was rising off a newborn calf's slimy body as her mother turned to meet and lick the calf's head.

There is something about these moments that anyone who observes them experiences: they bring joy, awe, and wonderment, even to a vet. I cleared the calf's nostrils of the birth liquid. The cow licked, thereby stimulating the newborn. One breath...another...the cow kept licking...another breath...relief and fulfilment.

'Thank you, Rob,' Jerry said. 'Can I get you anything?'

Snippets of a Vet's Life

'Perhaps a towel, and a warm cup of black coffee. But first, let's get them into a shed. Otherwise, the calf could still die.'

This was a good moment. I still had the knack with cows…just. And I felt good.

39 – CHADWICK AND CO

Max McClintock was on the phone.

'I'm sure you will be interested to know that I think the rodents are staging a siege. And even though I now have rodent-resistant bins, as you suggested after losing my mare to lepto, I can still smell their urine when I walk into the feed shed. Probably they've set up camp in the hay, and surprise, surprise, Wager is useless!'

'He's a foxhound, not a cat. What happened to your last cat? I think you said it went missing. I know you blamed Wager. Did it ever turn up?'

'It did, and the rats and mice were under control, but then it disappeared again one day, about two weeks ago, and about the same time, one of my agisters left. Anyway, that cat was useless. It was always trying to make friends with people, and it was afraid of your mate Wager, and was always trying to get into our house. Anne, in particular, didn't like it. She's NOT a cat person. Does that surprise you?'

I did not comment; instead, I said, 'I think you need another cat.'

Snippets of a Vet's Life

'Yes, my young friend. Thanks for the blatantly obvious. And do you possibly know where I can get one, a mouser, and not a little friend? But one who will survive this place and live in the feed shed, and preferably one who doesn't like people. I found more rat poo in the oats again this morning, even though there is a lid, and I'm worried that another horse might catch something, like Lucy.'

I gave him the name and phone number of the local animal refuge and thought no more of Max's need for a cat until a few days later, when I received another call from Max to report that a horse had a thick nasal discharge. I arranged to visit just after lunch.

As I parked my car, he came out of the stable.

'How's Wager?' A question that I always asked, and one which Max always responded with the same sardonic, and at times, slightly acerbic tone with the brief suggestion of a smile.

'You may well ask, my young friend. It was your Wager.'

'Not strictly, he's sort of yours now,' I reminded him.

'And for that gift, I am indeed always indebted, or not, hard to say.'

We entered the stable block, and I spied a large black cat sunning himself on the red brick floor at the far end.

'That's Chadwick, the new addition. He's not very personable, but I have found one or two dead mice on the floor over the last few days. Wager and Chadwick don't exactly hit it off. Does that surprise you?'

I let his question go through to the keeper, as they say in cricketing circles.

While Max held 'Sole Trader', a bay thoroughbred gelding, I took the horse's rectal temperature. It was elevated. There was a thick yellow discharge hanging from both nostrils, and signs of snot on the stable floor. I listened to the lungs and heart.

'When did this start?'

'About 2 days ago. Looking worse today, hence I thought I'd call out the 'viterinary', at great expense.'

'Does he belong to one of your clients?'

'No. He's mine. Left over from the interesting stage of my life, where Anne and I were members of a racehorse syndicate. Need I mention that it was Anne's idea?'

'Oh. How did that go?'

'How do you think?. Anne loved the races. Needed a new outfit every time one of the horses raced. I quickly realised that it wasn't the sure-fire way to riches that the trainer promised. Enough of that. Not my finest investment decision, but we did end up with this horse. Anne's idea. She felt sorry for him. And of course, being a thoroughbred means he's a bit mad. I can't ride him, so he just sits in the paddock eating the profits. Now he's sick, and you are here. So go easy on the bill! I expect the best of care at basement prices.'

'Of course, like you and most of the horse owners. I'll let Joan, the accounts lady at the office, know. Owned by a special needs client.'

He looked at me with that characteristic, slightly mocking, but slightly amused, look.

'Special needs, indeed, my young veterinary? Indeed.'

Over the time I had known him, Max and I had relaxed into a mutually respectful banter, which mainly revolved around the cost of my visits or the shenanigans of Wager, the old foxhound I had convinced them to take in.

'What do you think? Be alright?' Max asked with a concerned look, which for Max, was unusual.

'I think it's strangles.' I was referring to an infectious disease that had been the scourge of horses since the start of time, but was now treatable by antibiotics and could be prevented by vaccinations.

'Strangles! Isn't that contagious?'

'Yep. Very contagious. But luckily, it should respond to a course of penicillin injections, twice daily into his bum. Can you do that, if I show you how?'

'If it means saving money, yes, show me. Why not the neck? Bit safer for me.'

'Multiple injections into the neck often result in a very sore, infected neck, probably because as the needle goes through the skin, it takes a small section of the skin with it, and that introduces the bugs. So best to give them into the flank, high up, and alternate sides each time. Sure, you can do it?'

'Yep. Show me.'

I did. Max was similar to most of my clients. They became proficient over time at administering horse injections, especially the few trainers I worked with.

'I'll be back later this week to check, and we'd better make a day to vaccinate all of the horses for Strangles. I'll give you a cut rate, per horse.'

'Too kind,' was all he said as I left.

I dropped in a few days later and checked on Sole Trader. Max had done a good job of administering the twice-daily injection, and there was no nasal discharge. The horse's temperature had also returned to normal. He did have a slight cough, but that was not uncommon after a bout of Strangles.

As I was about to leave, Chadwick walked past me and flicked his tail against my leg. Automatically, I went to lean down to pat him, when Max said loudly, 'I wouldn't do that, my young veterinary.'

'No?'

'Don't be fooled by his apparent friendly demeanour. One of the new agisters tried to pick him up the other day, and I did warn her, but she said she had a special affinity for cats. Well, let me just conclude by saying that I had to take her to the doctor.'

'Any sign of rats or mice now?'

'None. Chadwick earns his keep, with no help from Wager!'

'How's he getting along with Wager? I hope the old hound isn't trying to catch the cat. It could be a bit messy if he did'

'Catch Chadwick! Doubt it. That cat has the agility of a gazelle, and Wager, the body of an old rugby player, and just as slow!'

'That's a bit unkind…'

'To Wager?'

'No. To retired rugby players.'

Over time, I realised that a system was in place. Not one that was written down, displayed on a whiteboard, or even explained to newcomers with an induction checklist. Max looked after the stables and collected the money from the agisters. Anne spent the money. Wager kept watch or slept. Chadwick ruled through fear.

It was like a modern-day Animal Farm, but without the betrayals.

And I was the vet. I arrived when called, drank whatever was offered afterwards, and left without disturbing the fragile yet oddly effective social and economic system that encompassed Max and Anne.

Snippets of a Vet's Life

40 – THREE LEGS, TWO FRIENDS AND ONE GOAT

'He's only got three legs, Rob!'

Victoria stood there, hands planted firmly on her hips, peering into the crate on the backseat of my car. Her tone said, 'You're joking,' but I could tell she was already half in love with the goat.

'But he is cute...' she added.

'He gets by,' I replied. 'You should've seen him at the clinic. Climbed a stack of hay bales like a rock climber on espresso. Three legs, no brakes, and zero fear.'

Tim squinted at the little animal. 'We're not running a rescue centre, you know.'

'No,' I said. 'But you've got paddocks. You've got Columbina. And most importantly, you've got kind hearts.'

Tim gave me the look he usually reserved for leaking pipes and the arrival of vet bills.

Kevin, the goat in question, was a bit of a miracle. Found tangled in barbed wire, one front leg so far gone that we either had to put him down or amputate the damaged leg. His owners, already had a horse that they couldn't really afford, and a first baby on the way. As much as they loved him, they could not afford the cost of the surgery, and so made the hard choice to end his life.

'Even if we could afford the surgery, I don't think we could keep him, with the baby on the way,' the soon to be young father said.

'We don't usually do this, but leave him with us. I may have a home for him.'

I felt sorry for the family and their injured goat, and it was a quiet day. So I operated.

Most animals would have curled up and retreat for a day or two. Not Kevin. After the surgery and a speedy recovery, he bounced back, literally. Loud, opinionated, and blissfully unaware of his limitations.

'He can't stay here,' Joan said after a particularly joyful romp through her office had knocked over the rubbish bin and a pot plant.

Joan was not a goat person, I discovered. Hence, I reached out to Victoria, who had agreed. I forgot to mention that Kevin lacked a right front leg.

I opened the crate. Kevin burst forth with the energy of a goat who didn't know he was missing a leg- and rammed straight into my shin.

Snippets of a Vet's Life

'See what I mean?' I said, steadying myself, and rubbing my injured leg. 'Confidence on hooves.'

Columbina was grazing under the fig tree and had turned to look. She began her slow, deliberate approach. I knew that look. She had sized up new chooks, rogue alpacas, even a drama student once, and now she was considering the goat.

Kevin saw her. He didn't shy away. He didn't bolt. He loped forward with the confidence only a goat can muster, gave a polite bleat, and stopped.

They stared at one another. Long and silent.

Then Columbina gave a snort, a dignified, matriarchal kind of snort, turned, and walked away.

'That's donkey-speak for "acceptable,"' Victoria translated.

Kevin followed her like he'd always belonged. I watched as he positioned himself beside her in the grass. She didn't protest.

'Well,' said Victoria, 'that was easy. And they'll be good for each other. He's got spunk. She's got wisdom. Together, they'll balance out.'

Tim grunted. 'So I guess that means he stays, then?' looking at his wife.

Kevin didn't just settle in, he took over. Within days, he'd learned the layout of the property, established dominance over the ducks, and figured out where Victoria kept the chook food. He had also developed an odd habit of trailing behind Columbina like a three-legged shadow, bleating his opinions on everything from sunrise to shovel handles.

He was clever, that goat. Too clever, if I were honest.

The trouble started with the laundry.

It was subtle at first. A sock missing here, a tea towel disappearing there. Victoria blamed the wind. Tim blamed Victoria.

Then one morning, I arrived to find Kevin dragging what looked suspiciously like a pair of underpants across the driveway.

'He's got a taste for cotton,' Victoria muttered, chasing after him with a broom.

It turned out Kevin had taken a liking to the clothesline, or more accurately, the laundry on the line. The end sections were within reach of a rearing goat with just the right amount of reckless energy and using a nearby tree stump stump that worked as a springboard.

I suggested moving the line. They tried. Kevin adapted.

He began climbing an another stump by the fence and launching himself into the air like some kind of acrobatic pirate. One memorable day, he turned up in the garden wearing Victoria's apron and a pair of Tim's socks around his horns.

'Do something!' Tim growled over the phone at me.

'About his fashion sense?'

'About his appetite for my wife's undergarments!'

'He's just expressing himself.'

But I got it. Not everyone appreciates a goat that treats the washing like a buffet. So I made some suggestions for curtailing his eating preferences.

They tried everything. Raised the line. Built a barrier. Even pegged a bar of soap as a decoy snack. Nothing worked. Kevin was determined, resourceful, and proudly unrepentant.

Then came the incident with the *note*.

Victoria had written a reminder for Tim. 'Feed Columbina before Rob arrives. Don't forget.' And she pegged it right next to the socks on the line.

But before it could be read, the note vanished. Kevin ate it, every last bit.

I showed up and found Columbina still unfed, glaring at the world with an apparent righteous indignation.

'You've made her grumpy,' I said.

'I never got the note,' Tim protested.

'I think Kevin ate it,' Victoria replied.

Kevin just stood nearby, chewing on a forgotten face washer, looking deeply pleased with himself.

In the end, Tim, using a certain flair, built a netted enclosure around the clothesline. It looked like a chicken coop designed by Salvador Dalí, but it worked.

Kevin moved on to new hobbies, mostly pestering the ducks and rearranging the chook feed containers, but occasionally, just occasionally, a rogue sock would still disappear.

And occasionally, when I would call, I would see him lying under the fig tree beside Columbina, half asleep, tail flicking gently, and a suspicious bit of pink elastic sticking out from behind the water tank.

'Some goats,' I commented, 'are just built to misbehave.'

Victoria didn't disagree.

Tim commented, 'Though he be but limping, he is fierce.'

'Socrates?'

'Nah. A Midsummer Night's Dream.'

Snippets of a Vet's Life

41 – DINNER AT THE GREEN COTTAGE

The Green Cottage had a way of looking more charming from the outside than it ever felt like to live in. When viewed from the Healesville road, it stood there like a postcard. A whitewashed cottage, green shutters, green roof, wild roses trained over the front fence, and bordered on one side by a hedge and a line of pine trees on the other. If being sold, an agent would probably describe it as 'something sturdy and well-loved, and in need of renovation.' But a closer inspection would have revealed what it was. A run-down wooden structure, standing on sinking foundations, and battered around the edges. It should have been demolished years earlier. Inside, the floors creaked, the kitchen sulked with its unreliable wood oven, and the whole place seemed to have been designed by someone who disliked right angles.

Still, it was my home, and I took pride in it.

It was also, on that particular evening, the stage for what I had rashly described to Max and Anne McClintoch as 'a little dinner at my place with some friends from University' Over the time I had known them, they had been generous in their friendship and had invited me to a few dinners. Wager would always greet me, and Max would make some remark about me dumping the old foxhound on them. Anne, in turn, would always complain about something that Max had recently done, but never severely. She clearly loved him. They were easy to be around. I wanted to return the favour, so I organised a dinner.

And I also invited two friends from my university days. Lachlan and Emma, his wife, had also asked me to dinner at various times, and it was time for me to return their generosity. They lived in the city, and their lives were in many ways different to mine. Lachlan was on track to become a specialist in Infectious disease, and Emma was a speech therapist. Since university and marriage, she had cleverly managed their joint incomes, so by the time of this dinner, they owned and lived in a good house, and in a good area. As she commented once, when discussing real estate investment, 'It runs in the family.'

As I quietly reflected, I was gradually falling behind. I was living in a ramshackle weatherboard cottage in the country, paying rent of a peppercorn a year. Such is life, and the cost of something that is *free*.

At the end of the phone call, Emma volunteered to bring her friend Judith, 'to round up the numbers,' she said, and then, perhaps sensing that I wasn't quite on board with this idea, added, 'I'm sure you will like her.

She's another speech therapist.'

I could hear the enthusiasm in her voice, so I agreed, 'OK,' and I resigned myself to yet another blind date.

There was a minor catering issue. Apart from white toast, I was hopeless in the kitchen. My last attempt at a dinner party, some weeks earlier, involved making 'Budget Beef Wellington' for the local farrier and his wife, followed by a sponge cake dessert. It might have been a bit ambitious, but I thought it sounded simple. Unfortunately, I misread the instructions, and when told to 'mix all the ingredients,' I did exactly that. Somehow, the cooking didn't go according to plan, probably because 'bake at 160 degrees' is hard to judge using a wood oven, and when I went to serve it, the sponge hadn't risen. Always the problem solver, I topped it with a can of peaches and called it a peach trifle. When I served the dessert, one of the ingredients, the bicarbonate of soda, remained under-cooked, and when eaten, and mixed with stomach acid, it released carbon dioxide, causing hiccups and belching. I understood the chemistry of cooking, but that didn't make me a cook.

So this time, a different plan. I outsourced dinner preparation to a lady who had recently started a business providing meals at home. It also helped that she was a horse owner and a client, and owed me money...the arrangement was a double win.

Max and Anne arrived first. Anne swept in with her usual brisk grace, the kind of presence that makes one feel as if she had been appointed chairperson of the room. Max followed, looking at Anne, and shaking his head at me in that quiet, jeering way he had perfected, as though he carried the permanent burden of being her minder.

'Rob,' he said, pausing in the doorway, 'it still amazes me that you managed to offload that foxhound on me. Wager! An animal that sheds more hair in a week than a barber's floor. And slobbers. Constantly. Anne assures me he's affectionate, but I think she means sticky.'

Anne rolled her eyes. 'Ignore him, Robert,' as she always called me, 'Wager adores him, though you wouldn't believe it from his tone.'

I grinned, half apologetic, half smug. As you know, Wager had indeed been my gift, or, as Max described it, my successful ambush and the old foxhound had needed a home, and Max, despite his muttering, was the sort of man who never truly said no to an animal in need. I had known that. He knew I had known that. And thus, the subject arose every time we met. It was an old joke that bonded us.

Emma and Lachlan arrived next. Lachlan was slightly older both than Emma and me, and they had met when the three of us were living in university colleges. After a quick romance, I read in the paper many months later that they were engaged. About a year later, they married. I was a guest at their wedding, and afterwards, we kept in contact. Lachlan, one of those men who was always confident with words, was sociable, well-liked and proud of his intellect. Emma was also an intellect, but there was something more... Emma glowed. She always had. There was something in the way she laughed, the way she turned her head to listen that made one feel she was lit from within. She made me, and others, feel included in her life. But she was married to Lachlan, which was the sort of cruel arrangement life seemed particularly fond of arranging for me.

I took her outstretched her hand, perhaps a fraction longer than was polite, and I think Anne noticed, because she gave me a look over Emma's shoulder that seemed to say, 'careful, Robert!'

Anne's glance was brief, but sharp. I was learning how much could be spoken without words: a raised eyebrow, a sideways smile. I knew that animals had their ways, a flicker of an ear, a twitch of a rump, and so did friends.

Finally came the arranged, blind date. Judith was perfectly pleasant, if a little intense. She asked questions as though taking notes for an exam: Did I enjoy being a vet? What sort of pets did I prefer? Have I ever considered leaving the profession? All this before I'd even taken her coat.

As we gathered in the sitting room, drinks were poured, and the conversation began its awkward, yet familiar, dance toward familiarity. I noticed, however, that the three women, Anne, Emma, and Judith kept glancing towards the kitchen. They were polite about it, but there was a question forming on their lips.

They thought they were discreet, but I caught the exchanged glances. It struck me that people were no harder to read than animals: you just had to notice what wasn't happening. In this case, the missing smell of dinner.

Finally, Emma, always polite, said it. 'Rob, what is that lovely smell?'

The trouble was, there wasn't one. The cottage smelled faintly of damp, mingled with smoke that had escaped the fireplace.

I cleared my throat. 'Ah… yes. It's subtle, isn't it? This oven is a wood stove, and cooking on it can be… temperamental. But, I have solved the problem in another way,' and left them with a slight mystery.

Anne raised an eyebrow. Emma exchanged a glance with Judith. Max, oblivious, was in the corner explaining to Lachlan how Wager had once chased the driver of a delivery van into the neighbour's orchard.

'Robert, are we all going out for dinner?' Always direct, this was Anne's way of addressing the question about the no-cooking odour.

I responded simply with a Cheshire cat smile.

Snippets of a Vet's Life

The minutes passed, the scrutiny deepened, and I began to feel the heat of my deception.

'Anybody for a top up?'

Would the knock at the door come at the right time? Would the meal be delivered before my ruse was exposed entirely? I imagined Anne marching into the kitchen, lifting lids and discovering only a cold oven and a pan of unused potatoes.

And then, salvation. A discreet tap at the back door, which I answered with the speed of a man fearing exposure. In came the trays, of roast lamb, vegetables, sauces, and all neatly packed and still warm. I thanked my client under my breath and whisked the lot onto the table with the air of a magician producing rabbits.

'Dinner is served!' I announced.

There was a moment of silence as they took in the spread, and then Anne said, dryly, 'Well, Robert, I must admit, I'm impressed. Not a pot out of place, not a dish left to soak. Remarkable.'

'It's my system,' I said, trying to look wise. 'Organisation, that's the key. A place for everything, and everything in its place.'

Emma laughed, and my heart lifted, until she reminded me that she was a vegetarian and didn't eat meat. Oops. I had forgotten.

Judith, however, was studying me with narrowed eyes, as if she suspected the presence of accomplices.

The meal progressed, course by course, as the conversation loosened with the wine flowing. Lachlan discoursed at length about a matter of medical politics. Anne, perhaps getting weary, tried to steer him towards lighter subjects, while Max muttered jokes under his breath for my amusement. Judith asked me whether I believed veterinary medicine was a calling or merely an occupation, which I parried by asking if she thought dinner was a hobby or a hunger..

Through it all, my attention kept drifting back to Emma. The way her hair caught the light, the way her eyes crinkled when she laughed at Max's dry humour. I found myself cataloguing the details, hoarding them, even as I knew they belonged not to me but to Lachlan, whose hand occasionally rested proprietorially on hers.

After the apple tart, Anne leaned back and declared the evening a triumph. Max agreed, though with a sly glance at me. 'Not bad, Rob. And all without a single trace of Wager's hair in the soup.'

The guests eventually left, coats gathered, and goodbyes exchanged. Judith pressed my hand earnestly, leaving me with the uneasy sense that she might expect a follow-up. Lachlan thanked me heartily, Emma smiled that smile that undid me, and then they were gone, leaving the cottage quiet again.

Snippets of a Vet's Life

I sat for a while in the empty dining room, the glasses half-drunk, the crumbs on the tablecloth. Outside, I heard a fox call.

The evening had been a success, at least by appearances. No one had gone hungry, no disasters had struck, and the Green Cottage had played its part. But as I cleared the plates, I knew that what lingered most was not the humour or the relief that the night went well, but the ache of something unspoken, the simple, impossible truth that I was in love with a woman who would never know. It was all a fantasy.

If I was learning anything as a vet, it was this: to pay attention to clues, however small. They told stories: about animals, and people.

Sadly, Emma gave me no clues. I was a friend to her, and nothing else, and I was just going to have to make the best of the situation.

Rod Graham

42 – THE CUT THAT DIDN'T GO TO PLAN

It was meant to be a routine gelding.

The sort of job you knock over before morning coffee, provided the colt is broken in and manageable.

We were in Max's back paddock, not far from Coldstream. The colt wasn't Max's. He belonged to one of Max's clients, a small-time breeder who'd asked Max to organise 'the snip.' Naturally, Max rang me.

'Quick and quiet,' he'd said. 'The owner wants to sell it as a gelding. Get a better price, he thinks. He's got a few people coming to look at the horse next week.'

Which is why, on a warm Tuesday morning, I found myself parked under a gum tree with my kit bag, surgical pack, and Wager the foxhound as always, in attendance.

Max had brought Wager along for the ride. He always did. And while he was meant to stay out of the way he had other ideas. He considered himself indispensable... Chief assistant to Max. Head of morale for Max. Keeper of unguarded sandwiches. Max kept saying how much he didn't like the dog, but the fact that Wager now travelled in the car with Max, and on the front seat, gave me some idea that things had changed.

Max, the good client that he was, had the colt waiting. The rangy, leggy youngster named Riffraff, was tied to the rail and looking deeply suspicious. I clipped a lead rope to the halter and patted his neck.

'OK. Nap, and then nip time.'

'You going to do it standing, or on the ground?'

He was referring to how many colts are castrated in the city stables, where it is not possible to anaesthetise them, so the procedure is done with the colt heavily sedated but still on its feet, and using local anaesthetic into the testicles to deaden the area, the chords are clamped with an emasculator before the testicles are quickly removed.

It's called a standing castration, and in skilled hands, it is a safe procedure and less traumatic for the horse. However, the trick is to have a skilled person holding the horse, always ready for the unexpected, such as a sudden kick in the direction of the vet. At times, I reflected that performing a standing castration was akin to being a veterinary thrill seeker.

Max, by his own admission, was still 'new' to the horse game, despite running an agistment business for horse owners for some time. I deemed it safer for Max, the colt, and me if I dropped the horse onto the ground with a short-acting general anaesthetic called thiopentone.

While Max held the colt's head, I injected a strong sedative into the jugular vein. After about five minutes, his head lowered, and his penis dropped out, which is a side effect of the tranquilliser. I quickly injected the dose of the liquid anaesthetic into the large vein in his neck and took the lead rope from Max.

'Just step back, Max. Sometimes they can fall forward in a struggle, or even plunge forward, as they lose control, and you can get injured.'

But not this time. The colt stood silently and then crumpled onto the ground as the bolus of drug hit the brain all at once. I rolled him onto his side.

'OK. Help me. I need assistance rolling him onto his back, and once he's in that position, I want you to hold him there by balancing him on his front legs. And quick, because we don't have a lot of time, four to five minutes, tops, before the drug starts wearing off and he comes out of it.'

For an older man, Max was quite agile, and for somebody who had been in management, he was able to take direction without question.

Years earlier, an old horse dealer had me out one day to castrate six of his colts. Before I arrived, he had negotiated a cut -price deal, but without letting me know that they were unbroken. Had I known, the price would have been more, because it is much harder to handle an unbroken colt. When I eventually got the first colt on the ground, I asked the old man to pull the uppermost hind leg forward so that I could reach over and remove the testicles.

'Nah, Mate. There's an easier way. Just roll the colt on his back, and the testicles will just pop up. No struggle.'

'Sure?' I had never heard of this technique.

'Done hundreds, matey, in the old days. Before you were probably even a glint in your father's eyes, I'm just getting too old, otherwise you wouldn't be doing this, and I would save myself a small fortune!'

We did as he said, easily placing the sleeping colt on his back, and as the old man balanced the upside-down colt by holding the front legs, and as predicted, the testicles popped up in the scrotum in an easy position to remove. And so the old man was correct. It was much easier to castrate them that way, and once again, I learnt something from a horse dealer.

Max did as I asked, and by holding the front legs, he was able to balance the sleeping colt on its back, allowing me easy access to the scrotum between the hind legs.

I got to work. Clean hands, no need for gloves... scalpel. I prepped the area with alcohol and moved quickly. An open castration is a straightforward procedure, but you don't want to hang about. Especially when your horse is upside down, and the anaesthetic is on a quick timer, and the horse will start waking up in a few minutes.

I clamped, cut, and dropped the first testicle into the kidney dish beside me.

That's when Wager made his move.

With the stealth of a fox and the enthusiasm of a Labrador, he darted forward, snatched the testicle from the dish, and took off.

'WAGER!' Max yelled.

'WAGER, NO!' I added, but could not suppress a laugh.

Too late. The hound bolted across the paddock, swinging his prize like a chew toy, ears flapping, tail high. Max looked as if he was about to give chase, but I stopped him.

'Leave him. No harm done. I need you to keep the colt on his back.'

I deftly removed the second testicle, crunching the cord closed and put it in the tray. Wager was nowhere to be seen.

'You know, I used to feel that. Whenever I crunched down on the cord, I felt it. Not now. You? Did you sort of feel it?'

'Veterinary, that's not fair. You won't get me to drop. I've been through much worse, in the army,' and I wondered what they got up to in the barracks.

Snippets of a Vet's Life

He looked at me with that typical Max half-smile when he was thinking something, but was not going to say anything.

'OK. Max. Let's move on. I've finished. Just lay his legs down, and then stand back. I'm going to keep him down for as long as possible by putting my weight on his neck. That's easy, but by the time I can't hold him down, the drug has mostly worn off, and he'll get straight up without struggle. OK?'

'And Wager, with the testicle?'

'Well. I've got no use for it. Have you? I'd give him the other one, but he probably won't need dinner tonight. Wager! Here, boy,' and the foxhound reappeared, and I threw him the second testicle. 'You know, Max, I have seen big grown men, and one, I remember, was a waterside worker, faint and collapse when I crunch down on the cord. You did well. The army was good training for you.'

'I must say, veterinary, that you did a good job.'

'And so did Wager! A good job cleaning up.'

He glared at Wager. 'He's still on probation.'

I looked at Wager. He blinked, yawned, and belched. The smell left no doubt. I turned to pack up the kit, glancing back at the colt, who was just beginning to twitch. It's always a critical time, that moment between sedation wearing off and full awareness returning. The horse can panic, struggle, or, worst of all, stagger to its feet before he is fully awake, and worst case, break a leg.

Max bent over to untie the rope from the rail when the colt gave a violent kick with his near hind leg, still recovering. Max yelped and staggered backwards, grabbing at his inner thigh.

'You alright?'

'Not sure. Something's... not right.' He limped to the fence, one hand clutching his groin. 'I think I've been gelded by proxy.'

I tried not to laugh. I really did. But the image of Max hopping in circles while Wager trotted proudly nearby with a bloodstained tongue was too much.

'You know,' I said, 'some blokes have sympathy pains when their wife is giving birth. You've just taken it to a whole new level.'

'I'm going to need an ice pack. And possibly a priest.'

Just another day in the paddock. As I loaded the last of the gear into the car, Max hobbled after Wager, who had clearly decided his work was done and was heading back to the house in search of further snacks. I started the car and rolled down the window.

'You want me to check your groin before I go?'

'Only if you bring sedation.'

Snippets of a Vet's Life

I left him to it. As I drove off, I caught a glimpse of Wager trotting along the fence line, licking his lips and pausing occasionally to inspect the gum trees for any more delicacies.

Just another Tuesday in the Yarra Valley. Another gelding. Another story. And one very satisfied foxhound.

43 – ONE CHRISTMAS EVE

'John's in the hospital, and I want you to examine him.'

'But Heather, I'm a vet'.

'I know. But you will tell me a lot more than these bastard hospital doctors have told me!'

I had met Heather and John many years earlier, first as clients, and then they became friends. They ran a successful saddlery shop.

John had a chronic lung condition that was gradually getting worse, and his stays in hospitals were getting more frequent and longer. I interpreted Heather's call for my assistance as an emotional cry for support.

And like my horse, Bos, Heather also owned a special horse, Miss Piggy. She was an equine flirt and a bit overweight; she could also be demanding and histrionic at times. Whenever she and Bos were together, they acted like young lovers. Bos would preen, standing tall with his ears erect and eyes glistening. She would nuzzle him, squeal, then kick him in the abdomen before running away. Perhaps she was hoping for more? I don't think she ever realised that Bos wasn't complete; he was a gelding.

I liked to believe that she liked him for what he was, and not for what he wasn't.

I walked into the hospital and greeted John. His colour was not the best, but he still had that welcoming look on his face and a slight smile. Heather had obviously told him of the ruse. I looked at his nurses' report sheet at the end of his bed, felt his pulse, put my stethoscope to his chest, looked under his eyelids, looked in his ears, and, after talking to him quietly, left.

'It worked!' Heather was ecstatic on the phone later.

'After you left, the head ward nurse came over and asked who you were. I told them that you were our vet, and I was worried about John and had asked you to examine him.'

I was intrigued. 'What did she say to that?'

'She asked me why I would get a vet when the best hospital staff and doctors surrounded John?'

And she told them!

'Because he will tell me more than anybody in this hospital has about John's condition.'

I could imagine it and felt a bit for the staff.

People do strange things and reach for strange solutions when they are stressed. But as Heather told me when I next saw her, from then on, the staff were eager to keep her up to date with John's condition.

Sometime later, many weeks after John had been discharged, Heather called me out for Miss Piggy. She was worried.

It was Christmas Eve, and Miss Piggy had mild colic. Miss Piggy, true to her name, had broken into the feed shed and munched on the oats. It must have felt like Christmas and mince pies for her. However, much like us, if we overindulge in mince pies, she too had to face the consequences. She had a stomach ache and was occasionally squealing and kicking at her abdomen.

Like all responsible horse owners, the family took turns to keep Miss Piggy moving so she wouldn't collapse onto the ground and roll. Rolling is often what horses do when they have intestinal pain, but the act of rolling can sometimes make a simple stomach ache into something much more serious: it can cause the intestines to twist, and only surgery or death will resolve the issue.

Vets, not many people know, are the only clinicians licensed to use death as a treatment, and this was an option.

I listened to Miss Piggy's heart. Her rate was about 70 beats per minute. Elevated but not serious. With pain, the rate goes up and then settles again. With a twist, the rate continues to rise. Miss Piggy's reaction to her abdominal pain was more than that of many other horses suffering colic and having the same heart rate. Her response was over the top.

Not long after I arrived, Miss Piggy kicked at her abdomen and then, with great drama, threw herself on the ground. And then jumped up, walked around a bit and did it again, with a dramatic crumple to the ground. I listened to her heart. Not too fast. I listened to the right side of her upper abdomen. Silence. Usually, there is a gurgle-gurgle sound every 30 seconds. Lacking this sound typically indicates that the intestines are not functioning correctly. The gurgling sound results from a mixture of fluid and fibre propelled by the large intestine's contraction and the opening of the ileocecal valve as the contents are squashed into the horse's caecum. Often, abdominal pain results from the gut's failure to propel the contents forward, and the resultant backup causes increased pressure within the intestinal system. Stretching the wall of the intestines is painful, and it is this pain that causes the horse to kick at its abdomen.

Severe pain causes rolling as the horse is trying to 'self-relieve'.

The basis of managing colic in horses is to control the pain so that the horse is less inclined to roll and lessen the risk of twisting the gut. In time, contents often move and the pain will diminish, but not if the horse's guts are already twisted, in which case the only treatment is urgent surgery, or vet induced death. The vet's diagnostic dilemma is to choose between simple colic, where pain relief alone will manage the situation, and colic due to a twist, where surgery is required promptly.

Miss Piggy continued to try to get down periodically, and it became increasingly difficult to stop her. Two hours after I arrived, her heart rate remained around 70 beats per minute, but her response to the painful episodes was becoming more dramatic. I administered more pain relief. Her heart rate stayed the same. Still, no gut sounds. She wasn't getting worse, but she wasn't improving, so I decided to do an internal examination.

I took my shirt off and put on an examination glove, and while John controlled her, I gently slipped my fingers through her anus, into her rectum and on towards her large intestines. To be a horse vet, you need to take, at time, necessary risks. Doing a rectal examination on a horse and not contained by a 'crush' is one of those times. I felt inside her, and just as I found her caecum on her right side, I felt her tense, and I quickly removed my arm and fell backward as she attempted to 'double-barrel' me with her hind hooves. The warning tensing of the rump muscles that I had learned over the years to respect meant that a horse was about to kick.

The first time I had felt it was my very first horse case. I was doing a pregnancy test via internal palpation of a mare's uterus. Not realising at that stage, the warning that it was, I took no protective action, and as Jane and Sonia, the owners of the mare, later told me, I went white in the face after the mare's hooves went on either side of my head.

Colics can often be all-night vigils, and the way Miss Piggy was reacting, this looked to be the case for this night. I had plans for the evening: it was Christmas Eve, but I couldn't leave Miss Piggy. The hours dragged on, and gradually, Miss Piggy became more violent, and it was harder to keep her walking. Occasionally, she was successful, and she managed to roll.

About 1:30 am, her heart rate was about 85 beats per minute, and she was sweating with the pain. Heather, not unreasonably, was getting concerned.

'She's going to die. I just know it.'

Over the years of our friendship, Heather, I realised, often took a more negative view of situations and people. It was just her style.

'I'm not sure,' I said, attempting to reassure her, but I was starting to wonder. 'I'm going to do another test to try to determine if she has twisted her guts.'

I sterilised the hair and skin under her abdomen and placed an 18 – gauge needle against her skin and, with a hard tap on the top of the 5cm needle, pushed it into her abdomen. A small quantity of yellow fluid came out. It was a good sign.

'OK,' I said to Heather. 'If she had twisted her gut,

there would be a lot more fluid coming out of the end of her needle. So, I don't think we are dealing with a twist. In addition, her heart rate is elevated but not excessively.'

'I don't want her to suffer. Promise me that if she gets worse, you will put her down. I can't handle this, so I am going inside and to bed.'

I knew that Heather loved Miss Piggy, and even though she sounded rational, I knew that she was very distressed. Going to bed was not a sign that she didn't care, but a sign that she couldn't handle Miss Piggy's distress. So, I gave Miss Piggy another dose of a strong painkiller and a drug to help her intestines relax and stop any spasms resulting from the pain.

There was a lull in her behaviour for about half an hour, and then her excessive physical reaction to the pain started again.

By 2:15 am, it was nearly impossible to stop her from throwing herself to the ground every 5 minutes. Even though she had a lot of medication on board, her reaction to the pain was not lessening, and she was becoming increasingly unmanageable.

Heather's request was at the back of my mind: 'I don't want her to suffer.'

Often, a colic presents end of life dilemmas for a vet. If a referral is not available, which can sometimes depend on distance or, more often, finances, then it is left for the vet to decide, to judge and to make decisions.

Snippets of a Vet's Life

There are some situations where the attending vet, having to act alone and with no other vet to help, is left with 'negotiating with God.' This was one of those situations.

Miss Piggy was apparently getting worse. She was getting more uncontrollable and hence dangerous.

Heather did not want her to 'suffer.'

I wasn't able to complete the internal examination of her abdomen. And I didn't have all the information that I needed to diagnose the cause of her pain. The pain appeared to be unresponsive to the medication.

John, who had been out of the hospital for the last few weeks, asked, 'What do you think?'

'I think we're going to have to put her down.'.

'Sure?'

'Um...No.'

'OK. Heather will understand.'

'First, I will give her some more pain relief, and we will see what happens over the next half hour.'

But there was no change. After one particular violent display of pain, I made a decision.

'I don't think we are getting anywhere, John. I think the kindest thing to do is to end her life. I'm sorry.'

Not many owners realise how emotionally draining a decision to end an animal's life is for a vet. The drain is not so much the loss of life, as it is when a person dies, but is it the 'right decision'? Is there something that could be done to fix the problem? Even though the horse vet may be surrounded by people connected with a horse, the decision to recommend death as a treatment is the vet's acting alone. Often, in the field, when dealing with colic cases, there are no other colleagues available for consultation. Additionally, the vet may not have all the necessary information to make a definitive diagnosis and make the 'right' decision.

It was time to end Miss Piggy's life. I had made the call. While John held her head, I inserted gently but quickly a large-bore needle into her jugular vein on the left side of her neck.

Getting a horse to drop quickly is essential; otherwise, it can become very excited and break away from whoever is holding it, making the whole procedure dramatic and stressful for all involved.

I made sure that the needle was in Miss Piggy's jugular vein.

John stood behind me, holding the other syringes, ready to pass them to me as I injected them into her. I connected the first syringe.

I paused.

And for once, I was affected by the emotion of what I was about to do. I thought of Bos and the antics that he and Miss Piggy would get up to. I reconsidered my decision. I reanalysed the limit data I had.

Snippets of a Vet's Life

Her heart rate was still only about seventy-five beats per minute. Her gum colour was normal, and there was no sign of a twist when I had put the needle into her abdomen.

And yet, she was getting very violent, but Miss Piggy was always known to be 'emotional.' My rational brain was telling me that Miss Piggy was not as 'sick' as she seemed. I was putting her down mainly because Heather had implored me, 'Don't let her suffer!'

I disengaged the syringe, pulled the needle out of her vein, and turned to John. 'I'm not doing it just yet. I know that she looks bad, but let's give her more time.'

'Are you sure, Rob?' John asked.

'I'm not, and that is why I want to give her more time.'

I have not often done reconsidered the decision to end an animal's life, but at the last moment I did this night.

Half an hour later, Miss Piggy stopped attempting to roll, dropped her head and started to eat. Her colic, from whatever unknown cause, had resolved. Half an hour later, she passed faeces, and her gut sounds returned.

I have never before or since had a horse in my care so close to death as Miss Piggy was that Christmas Eve. It was late, so I stayed the night and slept on the couch. In the morning, I got up early, went to her bedroom, and tapped on Heather's shoulder.

She looked at me with sad eyes until I said, 'She's OK. I didn't put her down. She recovered.'

As she processed what I had said, her face lit up, and she jumped out of bed and hugged me. And as she hugged me, she was crying tears of joy, and then quietly said,

'Thank you.' And hugged me again.

It was the best Christmas present for both of us that year.

44 – A SNAKE IN THE GRASS

A car pulled up, and out jumped an unexpected visitor.

'Tiger snakes and toddlers just do not mix, Rob!' she exclaimed as she strode through the gate. And then, in a lower voice, added, 'and by the way, your phone's not working. That's why I drove over.'

The phone! The weekend had been quiet. I left the saddle on the front verandah where I had been cleaning it, and went inside. I picked up the phone. She was correct. There was no dial tone. I was uncontactable.

'Don't worry, I think Tim has reported it.'

'Thanks.'

The local phone system, which I knew from experience, could be temperamental, especially after heavy rains. And that Spring, we had our fair share of unseasonably heavy rain, interspersed with warm days.

'So what's this about a snake? With the weather, I'm not surprised you are seeing a few.'

Victoria struggled to keep calm as she told me.

'In the chook pen, Rob. A tiger snake. Right next to the nest box. I nearly stepped on it. Columbina tried to warn me, but stupidly, I ignored her brays. But she was right!'

Victoria was a firm believer in the wisdom of the old donkey.

'I'm guessing you didn't offer it a cup of tea and a biscuit?' I asked, somewhat stupidly I reflected as I said it.

She ignored my attempt at levity and pressed on. 'It was thick. Like… a length of garden hose. And it hissed. I'm sure it hissed. I don't think I've ever heard a snake hiss before, but this one did.'

Victoria was clearly distressed about the encounter with the snake. I knew that there had been previous encounters with snakes. Columbina, to protect the complaining ducks, had once chased one away. It was part of living in the country. And, I remembered with a shudder the one I had nearly stepped on one evening, a few weeks after moving into the Green Cottage.

'You seem very distressed. It's unlike you.'

She was breathing heavily, and then, probably in an attempt to self-calm, rubbed her arms and then said, more softly, 'I know snakes are part of it all. But our grandchildren are coming to stay. You know how it is. Our Emily toddles around without a care in the world.

Snippets of a Vet's Life

If one of them got bitten...'

I nodded. 'And that'd be the end of visits for good?'

'Exactly, and I would never forgive myself!'

She sat down on the garden chair and unconsciously rubbed her thighs.

'I just don't want to give our children any more excuses not to bring the grand-kids. They already think it's a bit odd that we live out here. And I'm starting to feel guilty. My mother helped me with my children, and increasingly I think I need to help them, and I can't if we live out here. Nothing is ever said outright by the kids, but there's an undercurrent, if you know what I mean. If they hear about that snake! I don't think the grandchildren would be allowed to visit. Their parents are already halfway there. Their visits are getting less.'

This had been brewing for a while. I'd heard the tone in her voice a few months back, when she joked about needing a stair-lift for the old tractor. Or when she said Columbina would outlive them both. I'd smiled, as I always did. But she'd meant it. She had a concern about their future, as they both got older, and about coping with animals on the farm.

Now, with the snake scare fresh and her hands trembling just slightly, it was clear that she was worried, but not just about snakes.

'Have you spoken to Tim? About your concerns?'

She hesitated, then nodded. 'He knows. He's just

being...well, Tim. He talks about fate and how he thought he'd die on that patch of land with a hen under one arm and a glass of wine in the other.'

'Sounds about right.'

'But even he's starting to look at real estate in the suburbs. Secretly, of course. He closes the paper when I walk in.'

I smiled. 'He'll come round. He always does.'

'But what about Columbina? And Kevin? They're family. They're not show animals, Rob. Kevin's got three legs and a foul temper. And Columbina's... well, you know. She's a philosopher.'

'So do you need help re-homing them? I'll see what I can do.'

Which is how I ended up in Max's paddock, a day later, watching Wager dig holes in the dirt and preparing to plead a case to Max that I wasn't sure I believed in myself.

'Absolutely not.'

That was Max's answer before I'd even finished the sentence.

'You didn't even hear the complete pitch.'

'I heard enough. Dare I mention the word Wager? I don't need a goat with a limp and a donkey with attitude.'

'Columbina has wisdom, not attitude. And Kevin?

Snippets of a Vet's Life

Well, what can I say? Interesting? Has three legs, yes, but is very agile, and is great at eating and getting rid of wild blackberries. I see you've got a bit of a problem with blackberry bushes sprouting up.'

'Rob!'

'And the donkey is very clever. She once rescued Kevin from the dam.'

'That's not a skill I need around here.'

I tried another angle.

'The owner found a tiger snake in the chook yard. She's freaking out. Worried about the grand-kids. They've decided to move. It's the right thing, but it's hard. They're heartbroken, Max. Those animals mean the world to them.'

Max scratched at the back of his neck. 'You're playing the guilt card?'

'Just laying out the facts. You do have the space...and now that your kids have left home. Perhaps?'

He didn't say anything for a while. Wager came up and dropped something foul at our feet. Possibly once a shoe. Possibly not. Luckily, it wasn't a dead rabbit or cat.

'A donkey will scare the agister's horses. No, I don't think you can offload this problem onto us, veterinary.'

I knew that donkeys communicate differently from horses. Horses use subtle body language, while donkeys are more vocal and slower to respond to pressure. This can confuse some horses at first.

'Trust me, Max,' and he looked at me with a slight smile and a look on his face that I interpreted as, *I trusted you last time, and that's how we got Wager.*

'Huh! Trust you! This is not about trust, my veterinary friend. This is about you offloading a problem,' and then, after a pause, muttered, 'I'll think about it.'

Which, in Max-speak, meant 'probably yes.'

That's all I needed.

Two weeks later, Victoria and Tim pulled up in their ageing Subaru. In the float behind, Columbina looked out with her usual knowing expression. Kevin, bandaged and braced, stood beside her, wobbling on his three good legs.

'You sure about this, Rob?' Tim asked, his voice low, after I introduced him to Max.

'They'll be safe here. Max has the acreage. Underneath, he is a good and kind person, but he just hides it. Their foxhound, Wager, will not be thrilled, and there's a cat, Chadwick, that Kevin will have to negotiate around, but I think Columbina will quickly set the rules and boundaries. For everybody, including the humans!'

Snippets of a Vet's Life

He thought for a moment, probably reflecting on what I had said and not for the first time referenced Animal Farm.

'I have made the same observation, Tim. The only thing missing is the nastiness of the pigs when they became the overlords.'

Victoria took my hand. 'Thank you, Rob, for helping. We're not going far. Just closer to the kids and grandkids. But this...this is the hardest part.'

Columbina brayed softly, almost as if to say, 'Enough talk. Let's begin the next phase.'

And just like that, for Victoria and Tim, the old life closed behind them, and for Max, a new era began, with a donkey philosopher, a goat with three legs, a slightly annoying but loyal foxhound, a cat with a severe attitude problem, and about twenty horses, happily grazing in their paddocks, and Anne collecting the money.

Victoria and Tim called me occasionally to report and check in.

'The city suits us, though Tim claims that the pigeons on the apartment roof are plotting against him. He's teaching drama at a community centre and has already directed a version of King Lear set in a retirement village.'

'And you, Victoria?'

'I volunteer at a gallery and recently hosted a

workshop titled 'Sketching the Invisible,' adding that the workshop was inspired by Columbina.

'Of course,' I said, acknowledging that the old donkey still had a part to play in their lives.

They sounded happy. Adjusting. But older, perhaps frailer. Not the same as Broomhill, of course. But they still asked after Kevin, as if he were a naughty royal in exile, and their beloved Columbina, the donkey oracle.

'Do you really think she has wisdom, or is she, after all, just a donkey? And it was your interpretation that gave the impression that she has wisdom.'

'Still not a believer, Rob? Yes. She has wisdom...for those who believe,' and I could almost hear Victoria smile, knowingly, at the other end of the phone.

And we left it at that, and I settled back into the routine of practice and living at the Green Cottage.

But a change was afoot, my stars realigned, and within two years, I had married, sold the horse practice, moved to the city, started a small animal practice, and became the step-parent of three young children, and the husband of a very successful and assertive wife.

I wondered if Columbina knew? Silly thoughts for a vet.

Snippets of a Vet's Life

45 – THE PURSUIT OF HAPPINESS

Someone or something kicked me in my back. I woke up with one hand on the floor; the hand was preventing me from falling out of bed. I looked over. There were three young children, two medium-sized dogs, and one very new and attractive wife in the bed with me.

So this was marriage, I thought.

Later, I said, to my new wife, 'Look, Emma, I understand the young children, but the dogs. I'm a vet, and dogs in bed... well... It's just not on.'

She replied just as quickly, 'Well. They were here first.'

It was a logic I couldn't overcome, and still can't, many years later, when I now share the bed with no children, two different dogs, and the same wife.

So, how did this radical change of life happen for me?

What seemed sudden had been written in the stars for a long time.

'Not many men get to marry the woman of their dreams, but I have today, ' and the sound of women swooning followed my words.

But getting married to her was never a given.

We actually met by chance one evening, in the second year of my vet course at the University of Melbourne, at the Law Society cocktail party in the ground-floor Common Room of Ormond College.

That wasn't the first time I'd seen her. A few hours earlier, I'd walked into the gates of Ormond College with two mates, one of them pretty smashed. He'd heard about a party and reckoned we should check it out.

Why not. It was the week of the first term, of my second year at Melbourne Uni, and nothing was happening.

I'm not sure if we had any plan except to have a look, but as we made our way towards the large wooden front doors of the college's main building, a Scottish castle-type edifice, we heard the sounds of a party being held around the corner of a hedge.

Our drunk friend, true to form, pointed at the crowd of students and then lurched towards the gathering. We tried to restrain him, but Peter, a mate, perhaps the social opportunist, said, 'No. Let him go, and then we will follow as though we are trying to restrain him.'

I released my grip, and he fell towards the assembled

group, picked himself up, and stumbled on. By this entry, we joined a group of about 80, mostly students, having a drink on the front lawn. As we soon learned, it was a 'Fresher's Party', welcoming new students to the College. We should not have been there, and I was feeling a bit guilty, but Peter was clearly in his element and quickly had a glass in his hand.

At one stage, I was engaged in an intense conversation, as students often do, with someone about something that I have now forgotten, when my drunk friend, true to form, stumbled and fell over. I felt he was beyond redemption, so I kept my distance. However, his stumbling and the minor ruckus it caused resulted in many party-goers looking in his direction, as I did.

And that was when I saw her for the first time across the crowded lawn, just briefly, then the crowd reformed, and my view of her was lost. Just like that, almost in the blink of an eye, I was smitten. Big time.

Chance, I was to discover, had returned as a director of my life.

Later that evening at the Law Society, start of the legal year, cocktail party, held upstairs at the same college, we again used the charade of the drunk friend to gain unauthorised admission, I actually met her for the first time, and we talked, and talked. And then she and her drunk boyfriend left, and we left. I was smitten.

Perhaps I was delusional, but latter, before going to bed for the night, I wrote in my diary that I had met, that day, the woman I was to marry.

But she seemingly played hard to get, even though I never revealed the depth of my attachment feelings to her when we were both students.

I would visit her in her room in Women's College, and announce my arrival by a very polite, hence soft, knock on her door. She was by nature polite and engaging, and I was by training polite, and when I visited, we would have cups of tea and talk about light-hearted things. Years later, when we were married, she told me that she thought, when we were at university, that I was a bit of a nerdy guy, a good friend, but nothing more than that. When I met her, she was going out with John. They had been the classic childhood sweethearts, and John was sporty, confident, loud, full of energy, and very popular. I felt that he seemed to have every attribute that I lacked. She was also popular, and together they made a great couple. However, something happened, and the relationship came to an end. Not long after, Emma became engaged to Lachlan, a final-year medical student.

I was devastated. I read about their engagement on the local newspaper's social media page.

Their wedding was a grand affair, and I had received an invitation. She was unaware of my feelings for her as

Snippets of a Vet's Life

I sat in the pew, watching my fantasy life with her slip away.

Later, at the reception, I found myself sitting with her mother. I suspected she had some inkling of my unrequited love for her daughter. When I expressed anguish at what to do, she merely muttered, 'Perhaps you should just stick around. She is a loyal friend.'

My feelings for her never abated as the years went on, and I always had trouble forming relationships with others because, secretly, perhaps unconsciously, I was constantly comparing a new partner with her. Gradually, she came to sit on an insurmountable pinnacle.

I was friends with the newly-married couple, and Emma would contact me for help whenever they moved homes. She proved to be good at selling and buying houses, and in time, they were able to move into a grand house, in a grand suburb, and in so doing became more out of reach for me, living in the country, for a peppercorn a year, in the ram-shackle Green Cottage.

And later, adding to the 'distance', three children arrived, and because now Emma considered me a close friend, I visited her in the hospital not long after the children were born: a girl and, two years later, a twin boy and a girl.

Their family was complete, and to any observer, they appeared to be a perfect couple.

However, after two years in the USA, they gradually moved, emotionally, in different directions, and one day, when they returned to Melbourne, they separated. This happened a few months after they had moved into a new double-story house, and as had previously happened, Emma asked me to help them move in. Lachlan, a newly minted medical specialist, was busy with work, so Emma and I did the job.

As we worked, I perceived a change. Nothing was said. Perhaps, unconsciously, she saw me in a different light. Perhaps unconsciously, I was now more than a good friend. On the way back to the Green Cottage later that day, I could not get the change out of my mind. Maybe it was how she held my hand as we crossed a road, but whatever it was, I felt that our friendship was different.

Eventually, I suggested that we spend more time together, and we did. However, it was too soon after the breakup, and she wasn't ready for a serious relationship. When she told me, I felt crushed once again.

In the fullness of time Emma consulted a fortune teller.

'There are two men in your life. One…it is passed. The other, a fair one, is deeply troubled and needs much work.'

This did not help my cause, but we continued to go horse riding in the country on weekends. We were members of the same horse riding club, which I had started with a few friends a few years earlier.

It was an emotionally challenging time for me, and perhaps for her as well. However the situation came to a head one Saturday night. I had proposed to her about a week earlier but received no definite answer.

A riding club dinner was to start in about an hour, and after some heated words, I announced, 'By the time we sit down for dinner, I need an answer. And to be frank, I have come to terms with the answer going either way. Either yes or no, but I need an answer. I cannot cope anymore with this indecision. If there is no answer, within the hour, I will take that as a,' and I paused as I realised the magnitude of what I was saying, 'as a no.'

The words were hard to say, but I had to know.

As we walked towards the dining room door, and true to her spontaneous, casual nature, she said, 'Yes.'

In the months that followed, while we were officially engaged, we built a house in the Yarra Valley, but it didn't turn out to be our home.

A year later, we were married at her home in the city, surrounded by many of her friends and a few of mine. And as I said the long awaited words, 'I do,' I had no idea how much my life was to change.

But Joan did. 'Do you think you can handle all of this, Boss?' she said, making an unspoken reference to the grand house, the three young children, and a successful, opinionated woman about to be my wife.

'Sure,' was my quick response.

'We shall see…'

A harbinger of the changes that were about to befall me occurred on the way back from our honeymoon. The three days spent away in the mountains, to be our time as newlyweds, ended in an argument. Some car rides are filled with noise, while others are filled with meaning unspoken. There was a deafening silence as we returned to the city. Ever the peacemaker, I thought about how to break the impasse and the silence. Eventually, I proffered what I judged to be a safe question.

'When are you selling the house in the city and moving into our home in the Yarra Valley?'

'What do you mean, sell the house in the city?' was her short response, not in the warmest tone.

The silence continued as I considered what to say next. Surely we had discussed where we were going to live, and the evidence for that was clear: the house we had just built in the Yarra Valley. I asked what I thought was the obvious question. 'Well, what about the house we have just built?'

I considered that there was no answer to that…but there was.

'I told you not to do that,' she shot back, quickly.

Snippets of a Vet's Life

Again, silence descended as I considered that during the building of the house in the Yarra Valley, if Emma had mentioned that she thought it was unwise for us to build a house, I would, for sure, have picked up on the comment and asked more. However, to this day, I have no memory of her bringing up the issue during our engagement.

That is how I moved to the city.

That is why, each morning for the next five years, I would drive to the Yarra Valley. Then, after work each night, I would drive the hour back to the city, my new home, and my new, instant family. And that is how the house in the Yarra Valley became, for a time, during the work week, the office for my horse practice, and at the weekend, a retreat for the family, and a place for the children's ponies.

Those magical words: "I do" caused my life to radically changed: a mortgage, added living costs, a ready made family, a lovely wife, and a new home address. All this required me to work harder and smarter. That is, until one day, we had a new plan.

We would establish a new clinic near our city home, sell the horse vet practice and the country house, which was now our weekend residence, and simplify my life in the process.

Or so I thought, at the time.

We eventually, months after an exhaustive search, found something suitable near our inner-city home, and

Emma and I renovated the old wooden building and once the permit arrived, opened for business. I now owned, not only a horse practice 59 minutes away from where I lived, but also a small-animal clinic about 5 minutes from where I lived, and my life became exceptionally complicated, with frequent back-and-forth trips between the city clinic and country office, always in a rush, and often running late.

This was years after the halcyon days at the Green Cottage, but back then even that arrangement had changed quickly.

One day, years earlier, and as I was paying for petrol in Coldstream, the proprietor, Ken, happened to say, 'I hear you're leaving.'

'What do you mean, Ken? Leaving what?'

'She was in here the other day, wondering how to get rid of you.' Ken could be straightforward sometimes, in a laconic country mechanic's way.

'Oh,' I said. 'Have I done something to upset her?'

'No'

'What then?'

'Can't say.'

'Thanks, Ken.'

Two days later, I received a note from Mrs Pridham requesting that I give up the Green Cottage. She was reviewing her estate, in preparation to transferring

Snippets of a Vet's Life

Emmerton House to a charity and knew that the cost of proper upkeep would be a financial drain and so demolition of the Green Cottage was arranged to prevent squatters in the meantime from taking up residence and thwarting her plans.

But, as it turns out, Mrs Pridham changed her mind and retained control of Emmerton House until her death, and then her heirs converted the stable block and old garage into a restaurant and reception centre, and on occasions, the main house was open to paying visitors in support of one charitable cause or another.

A few years after moving to the city, by chance, I saw her at a charity film night in Healesville. It was to be the last time. I was there with my wife. We had travelled from Melbourne, and I was excited to see my old friends from my Yarra Valley days, and as I entered the room, I saw her.

She was standing in a small group of older people. She looked frail and was slightly stooped. I approached and introduced my wife. She hesitantly smiled out of politeness, but I could see that she was confused, and she didn't seem to understand what I was doing or who I was.

'Mrs Pridham, I was your tenant. Do you remember me...the vet?' However, there was no recognition, and in confusion, her eyes darted away, as I nervously continued.

'I used to live in the Green Cottage, and we used to

talk about your chickens and one day we discussed the old lady in the hunting print, and you got a shock...and I wrote to you about the bell chimes and you wrote back. Do you recall?'

She looked at me with a distrustful stare. I could see that she couldn't remember. She looked away, uncomfortable, uncertain and flustered.

'I don't know you,' she quietly said, looking at me warily, excused herself, and wandered away.

On the way home later that night, we drove past where the Green Cottage had once stood, and it was as though none of what I remembered had ever happened.

The side hedge had gone.

The tall back trees had gone.

The big green gates that guarded the back entrance to the main house were gone.

The squeaky front gate had gone.

The Green Cottage had been demolished, and the land returned to the pastures from whence it had come.

All had gone.

Except for my memories, this long tale, and an old hand-coloured hunting print called 'The Heythrop Hunt.'

46 – THE LAST CALL

'Hey, Boss,' Mike said, and I quietly wondered if this was the last time he would call me by this title. Mike was a relatively new graduate whom I had been successfully working with while I dashed between clinics. As many young graduates did, he left after a year and worked in England for a while, and then returned to settle down.

We caught up, and over lunch, he and I negotiated the sale to him of my horse practice.

A few weeks later, I was busy moving out of my office downstairs in the Old Cheese factory, when I heard him call out.

'Yes, Mike.'

'Are you still registered to do racehorse identification blood work?' He was referring to a system where every racehorse had to be identified via its blood and markings on its coat.

'Yes. I am. Your registration hasn't come through yet?'

'No. I was a bit slow in getting the paperwork done, and I know you're leaving. Could I get you to do one last call? The trainer sort of asked for you anyway, mate.'

And that is why, as I reflected, it was to be the last time I parked outside Jerry Treloar's stables in Yarra Glen. Jerry had been a struggling owner-trainer, and over the years, been the proud owner of one or two racehorses. He was what I would call a 'battler.' He lived for his horses, and I would sometimes see him at the local racetrack early in the morning, up on a horse doing his own track work. As he got older and heavier, it became harder for him to jump up onto the horse, and in time, he paid one of the local apprentices to exercise his horses.

Earlier in our parallel careers, he had called me to the track one morning because one of his horses started slobbering after an accident in which the horse had stumbled on its way off the track. The jockey had been propelled over the horse's head, reins still in his hands, and this had the result of pulling the bridle off the horse, and the horse had galloped away. Eventually, they were able to capture the horse and return it to the anxious Jerry. That is when he noticed the excess saliva from one side of the horse's mouth. He called me to have a look.

I put a mouth gag on the horse and opened his mouth. Inside one cheek was a long internal gash, probably due to the bridle and bit being forcibly removed from the horse's mouth as the jockey had flown over the horse's head, landing on the ground.

Snippets of a Vet's Life

'Oh. I bet that is sore, Jerry, and it explains the saliva,' I said as I pointed to it. 'Imagine if that was in your mouth. I'm not surprised he's drooling. Luckily, I can't see any broken teeth.'

'Bad? He's in a race this weekend. Do you think he'll be OK by then? I hope so 'cos I've set him up for this one...' and once again I reflected that horse racing is an industry based mostly on 'hope.'

'Not sure. It would be painful. You may have to scratch him from the race.'

'Can't....' and he looked at me as though there was more to his response.

'Can't?'

'Won't. He's been set for this race, but I can't say more. Mates have put a lot on his head. He's a long shot, but he's got a big, big chance. You should think about a bet.'

'Thanks, but I don't bet. If he has to race, for reasons I don't quite follow (and inwardly I was thinking there was something perhaps a bit 'dodgy' about the upcoming race) there is a new treatment that I saw at the last Horse Vet Conference. It's called Lotagen and works by removing dead tissue and allowing new healing tissue to form, quicker. It's the best I can offer.'

'Great! Let's do that.'

I applied some of the liquid to a cotton ball and placed it inside the horse's mouth. The damaged tissue turned white in response.

'I'll leave the bottle with you, and you apply it twice daily for the next three days. Stop using it by Thursday morning, and hopefully, it will be healed enough that he won't notice it when you put the bit in his mouth. Meanwhile, no ridden track work.. Get one of the pony boys to take him around the track on a lead. OK?'

'Sure. Whatever you say, Doc.'

'I should check him before he races.....'

'Nah. He will be OK. Also, got to save on expenses for a bit...vet bills. You guys aren't cheap. By the way, once we win, I'll be able to pay the bill...bit short this week.'

This request was not uncommon among the 'racing fraternity,' as this collection of often battling owners was sometimes referred to in the newspaper.

'OK. Good luck on the weekend. But, on the off chance that he doesn't win, do you think you could stump up some money now to pay the bill? There is an outstanding account as well.'

This was a strategy that Max McClintock, my long-time friend and long-suffering owner of Wager, the old foxhound, had worked out as a way of at least getting something at the time of service. Often it did work, but not this time.

'Mate. I want to, but as I said, a little light.... this

week. The wife is getting a bit funny again about the horses. And, it's her birthday…I guess I have to buy her something. But, don't worry, he's a cert.'

This was a new return strategy, I mused, blaming the wife for being short of funds.

'I'm not sure…'

'She'll be right, mate. The horse is a dead cert. Trust me.'

And again, I was left with the impression that there was something 'dodgy' in the pipeline. As much as he implored me 'not to worry', I was worried because receiving payment for horse practice in a timely fashion was an ongoing problem. The outstanding debt was gradually getting bigger, and Monday morning calls from the local bank manager were becoming more frequent.

As it happened, and totally unexpected by the bookies, which explained the very long betting odds, his horse did win the race on the following Saturday. The odds were very long, and from what I heard at the track the following week, Jerry had won a huge amount of money. It was rumoured to be thousands. And, as promised, Jerry did settle his outstanding account with us.

And something else happened that was completely unexpected. I was contacted by a few trainers, some of whom had not used me before, to get a bottle of the 'magic lotion' as one of them described it. Lotagen, the healing medicine I had applied to the inside of the horse's mouth, and then left with Jerry to use, was now famous at the local track, and everybody wanted some of the magic elixir that gave Jerry's horse the 'edge.'

The first trainer who called, looking to get some of the 'stuff' that Jerry used, did not believe me when I attempted to explain to him that Lotagen would have made no difference to the horse, and that 'he won on his merits', as they say.

'Nah. I want some. Can't say why. Can you give me a bottle?'

I reiterated that it wasn't a 'make them go faster' elixir, but an agent that debrided, or removed, damaged tissue.

'You're the vet, but I've seen it with my own eyes. Jerry's horse…WON'

I gave up.

That monetary windfall changed Jerry's future. He moved up in the local racing world. He quit his job working for the local shire, registered as a professional trainer, and in months had a small string of young horses to train. And since he attracted better quality horses, he started winning races, which had the effect of attracting new owners, and more importantly, owners who could afford to pay for better, quality horses.

Such are the vicissitudes of the racing industry.

So, this was to be my last job as a horse veterinarian.

Snippets of a Vet's Life

I parked outside 'Lotagen Lodge' as I always secretly called his stable and yard, grabbed my bag and walked into the stable. Jerry was busy with an owner and directed me towards a teenage girl.

'Cheryl, hold the 'Black Friday' colt while the vet IDs him and takes some blood. Think you can do that? And Doc. She's new but good.'

He then dismissed us and continued his conversation with the owner.

Cheryl held the black colt in the stable lane-way as I made notes about its markings: the left fetlock was white, two hair whorls adjacent in the centre of his head, above the level of the eyes, a few white hairs on his right rump, and nothing else. It wasn't much, but it was probably enough to identify him. I drew the markings on the identification sheet.

'OK. Now we need to get some blood. For safety, Cheryl, I think we should do this in a stall.'

Cheryl opened the stable door, and we both stepped in like it was any other day. The yearling colt followed, and as Cheryl turned back towards the stable door, the colt also turned around, and his rear end faced in my direction.

Then came the scream.

From Cheryl, a loud, sharp, and distinctly human in distress sound. She had caught her finger in the latch. At the same time, she let go of the lead rope. The colt reacting to the scream and confusion backed away from the gate, straight towards me.

I retreated to the far corner like a man who suddenly remembered he had somewhere else to be.

'Grab the rope! Pull him forward,' I shouted, trying to make my voice sound confident and not at all like someone cornered by a panicking half-tonne yearling.

Too late.

He lined me up. I saw his rump lift, that familiar gathering of equine muscle and bad intentions. I knew that posture. Every vet does. It's the horse equivalent of a bowler winding up a cricket ball, and I was the stumps.

I dropped to the corner. Flat to the straw, arms over my head, heart trying to get out through my ears. There was a heavy thud as his hoof slammed into the wall just above where my fragile head had been moments earlier. A polite warning shot, really.

I stayed down a beat longer than necessary, just to confirm I was still alive. Then I peeked up, and Cheryl had managed to grab the rope again, nursing her bruised finger. The colt stood blinking, the picture of innocence.

'You all right?' she asked as she pulled the colt's head towards her and rump away from me.

'Just re-evaluating my career choices,' I said from the floor, making fun of the situation to ease the tension, but in reality, it was the truth.

'That was close. I'm so sorry,' she said.

'No problem. How's your finger?'

I composed myself and got the two samples of blood from the colt's jugular vein, and then we exited the stall, leaving the colt to his own dark thoughts.

Jerry was still busy with his client, so I waved him goodbye.

Driving the way back to the clinic, for once, I wasn't in a rush. I had sold the horse practice. It wasn't my responsibility anymore. The day had no urgency. As the car rattled over the old timber bridge, as I left Yarra Glen, I noticed the sound of the loose planks clattering under the tyres, a noise I must have heard a thousand times but never truly registered. Today, the bridge spoke to me.

With no clients waiting, I let the Yarra Valley unfold around me. The paddocks, quietly green. A few horses lifting their heads as I passed. Cows bunched under a stand of gums. The road curved gently left, and in its centre, a rabbit, flattened but strangely intact, as if still in mid-leap. I slowed, not from necessity but from instinct. There was something almost solemn about that dead rabbit, its life snuffed out in an instant.

Something oddly familiar, but long forgotten.

And then I remembered my first call, years ago, just weeks into the job with Doug, my first and only veterinary boss. A pregnancy test for a mare named Dorothy, owned by two good women whose friendship had gradually faded. What hadn't slipped was the image of the mare's hind hoof flashing past my ribs, and how close I came to being kicked into the next life.

Funny what anchors us. I'd driven this route more times than I could count, always chasing the clock to get to the next client on time. But today, I finally saw it. The land around me. The friends who had sustained me. The beauty I'd passed without seeing. And the dead rabbit, in its way, reminded me where it all began, and I reflected on how quickly it had all gone.

And there was one final reflection: for the first time, I had been scared when the colt had me in the corner. I had been in many perilous situations involving horses over the years, but I had never been scared. So...it was time, and I finally knew it. As I passed through Coldstream, I saw a rubbish bin. I parked the car, and from the car's boot, I retrieved my trusty rubber stomach tube. As I walked towards the bin, I mused that I had used this stomach tube for many years. It was perhaps the first item of equipment I had purchased when I started on my own as a horse vet. I had used it countless times, and over the years, it had lost its bright orange colour. It was, in a way, the badge of being a horse vet. Symbolically, I put it in the bin and left that life behind me.

Snippets of a Vet's Life

Epilogue

This maybe the end of the book, but it is not the end of Snippets of a Vet's Life...to be continued.

For more information visit: vetsnippets.com.au

www.ingramcontent.com/pod-product-compliance
Lightning Source LLC
Chambersburg PA
CBHW020514080526
44583CB00013B/599